THE GRACIE DIET

"As a follower of the Gracie Diet from a young age, I can say that it is one of the most incredible health initiatives that the unpretentious Carlos Gracie presented us with so many years ago. Using his friends and family members as test subjects, Carlos developed a way of eating that optimized health and vitality. Rorion has done an amazing job providing readers with an insightful look into the principles and philosophy of this revolutionary diet while remaining absolute faithful to their origins. This is an incredible diet that has been refined by an incredible family over three generations. With this book, it is finally available for all to enjoy."

– João Alberto Barreto, *Jiu-Jitsu Grand Master, M.S. Clinical Psychology*

"The Gracie Diet is one of the most important factors in maintaining my health. Based on my personal experience, I know that if you eat purposefully, practice moderation in everything you do, and follow the guidelines in this book, I guarantee you will live a long happy life."

– Professor Pedro Sauer

"Some people claim that it takes at least forty years to evaluate a diet. The Gracie family has followed this diet for over eighty years – with impressive results. Our parents were healthy well into their 90's. All of our family members, students, and friends who have followed the Diet are models of health and vitality. We do get sick occasionally, but not very often and, so far, have never suffered from a serious illness. This leads me to believe that the Gracie Diet may not be perfect, but it is very close."

– Carlos Gracie Jr.

"I started the Gracie Diet at about 45 years of age and honestly feel as good as I did in my 20's. The Gracie philosophy has had an incredibly positive impact on my life."

– Jim Lona, *Government Sales Manager*

"In order to maximize your efficiency on the mat, you must also maximize your efficiency off the mat. The Gracie Diet is the secret to success."

– Ryron Gracie

"Growing up on the Gracie Diet was an incredible experience. From the very beginning, every food had its purpose and every meal had meaning. As a child, learning only to eat at designated times and to properly combine my foods gave me a level of discipline that became the driving force behind every one of my accomplishments, on and off the mat. I am forever in debt to the first and second generations of Gracies for developing a system of self-defense to which I could dedicate my life, but more importantly, for showing me the secret to a long, healthy and energetic lifestyle. I am eager to have children for many reasons, but none so much as to ensure that I can pass on the tradition of healthy living to the next generation of Gracies."

– Rener Gracie

"Carlos created a spectacular way of eating. If all Brazilians followed it, we would all be supermen."

– Jose Geraldo, *Journalist/Writer*

The Gracie Diet is simply sensational. I adopted the Diet in the 70s when I started training jiu-jitsu. To this day, the Diet keeps me fit, energized, and allows me to train every day."

– Professor Romero "Jacare" Cavalcanti

In the past, I tried several diets but never stuck with any of them because they were so restrictive. With the Gracie Diet, I get to eat all my favorite foods as long as I follow the combination guidelines and correctly space my meals. It's simple, it works, and I love it!"

– Eve Torres, *WWE Diva*

When I started training Gracie Jiu-Jitsu with Grand Master Helio Gracie and his sons, not only did it change my life in terms of self-confidence, discipline, and respect, but it also had a profound impact on my health. When I adopted the Gracie Diet, I was cured of hepatitis A in record time, and I finally came to understand that you really are what you eat. More than ever, Americans need to improve their health, making the Gracie Diet an invaluable asset for all of us."

– Professor Carlos "Caique" Elias

My greatest challenge was overcoming the fear of losing energy as a result of not eating for 4-5 hours. That fear quickly faded when I found that spacing my meals and mixing foods properly actually increased my energy and caused me to feel great all day long!"

– Ashkan Seyedi, *Computer Hardware Engineer*

We started the Gracie Diet before we were born! As soon as our mother became pregnant, our dad made sure that she only ate according to the principles of the Gracie Diet to ensure that we were growing in a healthy habitat. From birth, our parents taught us that nutrition plays a vital role in our health and that we should select and combine our foods in a rational way. Grandmaster Helio Gracie inspired us to cultivate the habit of "only eating what is good for you," and to reject the accepted norm that it is "ok to eat unhealthy foods once in a while." This discipline gave us the character and confidence to avoid soft drinks, candy, and junk food as children and alcohol and drugs later in life. Our unique diet disciplined our lifestyles. It not only shaped our minds and bodies, but also strengthened our family bond and inspired us to dedicate our lives to the dissemination of this philosophy through our Jiu-Jitsu schools."

– Valente Brothers

Through proper food combining and meal spacing, the Gracie Diet facilitates digestion and helps maintain the body's alkalinity for optimum health. Rorion Gracie is the right person to write this book. Not only does he have extensive knowledge of the Gracie Diet, but he has always strictly followed the concepts."

– Carla Gracie

THE GRACIE DIET

What Grand Master Carlos Gracie Discovered About Eating
After 65 Years of Research and Experimentation

Rorion Gracie

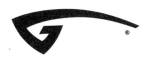

Gracie Publications

Library of Congress
Gracie, Rorion – The Gracie Diet

PCN Number: 2010915389

ISBN: 978-1-4507-4155-2

Gracie Publications
3515 Artesia Boulevard
Torrance, CA 90504 - USA
www.GracieAcademy.com
www.GracieDiet.com
www.GraciePublications.com
www.GracieUniversity.com

Printed in the USA

To Uncle Carlos

CONTENTS

PART ONE – THE GRACIE DIET

PART TWO – USING THE GRACIE DIET

FOREWORD

When I was a boy, the fighting arts always fascinated me. I wanted to learn to fight from the best. So, one day, when I was thirteen years old, my father, Dr. Syllo Valente, took me to the original Gracie Jiu-Jitsu Academy in Rio de Janeiro, Brazil, where he was already a student. There, I learned the techniques of Gracie Jiu-Jitsu from Grand Master Helio Gracie and, over time, became a competent practitioner of his family's art. From the moment I became a student at the Gracie Academy, I fully expected to learn the world's most effective fighting system, but what I never foresaw was that the fighting art's accompanying philosophy would transform, not only my life, but that of future generations of my own family. From that Gracie "blueprint for life" I learned that food and sex were not merely sources of pleasure, they were also a means of improving the overall quality of life and procreating. I also learned that by fasting, combining foods properly, spacing meals correctly, choosing the right partner, practicing good hygiene, working hard, and courageously defending truth and justice, I was better prepared to face and overcome many adversaries that so often overcome humans, such as disease, fear, and cowardice.

A core component of the Gracie family's philosophy was the "Gracie Diet," known in Portuguese at the time as "Regime de Alimentação Racional" or "The Rational Nutritional Regimen." This nutritional regimen is a result of 65 years of research and experimentation by the late Grand Master, Carlos Gracie. He based his diet on eating natural foods and combining them in ways that would allow for efficient digestion to promote optimum health. The 18th century French chemist, Antoine Lavoisier, established the doctrine that "life is a chemical function." Based on this principle, the Gracie Diet presents food combination guidelines designed to prevent unhealthy chemical reactions in the digestive process such as fermentation and acidity.

When I graduated from medical school in 1963, I decided to dedicate myself to the study of nutrition, in addition to my specialization in plastic surgery. I was the first physician to prescribe the Gracie Diet to patients during their pre- and post-surgery periods in order to speed their recovery. At that time, Grand Master Carlos Gracie would frequently visit me at my clinic to discuss my observations in order to improve our practices. We continued this exchange of information and experimentation until Carlos passed away in 1994.

I still apply the Gracie Diet, not only with my patients, but also with professional athletes. Recently, I introduced the principles of Carlos Gracie's diet to one of the world's most famous soccer clubs, Brazil's Vasco da Gama. Soccer legend Romário credited the Gracie Diet for his unprecedented feat of winning the Brazilian Soccer League's scoring title at the age of 40 in 2006. A couple of years later, Romário scored his 1000th goal, a mark only achieved by Pelé, the greatest soccer player of all time. The Gracie Diet also played a significant role in the education of my four children. My three sons, who run the Gracie Jiu-Jitsu Academy in Miami, have strictly followed the diet all of their lives as well as avoiding drugs, alcohol, and cigarettes. My daughter, Joana, is an internationally acclaimed show jumping horse rider and attributes her success in part to the health benefits promoted by the Gracie Diet.

In 1978, Helio Gracie's oldest son, Rorion Gracie, journeyed to America with the unwavering objective of teaching Gracie Jiu-Jitsu to the world. It was such a monumental endeavor that even his closest friends thought it an impossible task. With technique, vision, and relentless determination, he not only achieved his goal but surpassed everyone's expectations. Now, he is about to embark on an even more ambitious venture – to improve the world's health by sharing the benefits of this incredible diet. My hope, for the sake of everyone's health, is that he succeeds again. I believe he will.

Pedro Valente, M.D.

INTRODUCTION

I came to America in the 1970s with a single objective – to establish my family's Brazilian style of jiu-jitsu as the most effective self-defense system in the world. To prove my point, I challenged anyone – regardless of size, weight, athleticism, or martial arts skill – to defeat me in one-on-one, no-holds barred combat. I quickly convinced the martial arts community in Southern California that the Gracie system was amazingly effective. In 1993, I co-created the Ultimate Fighting Championship® to showcase my family's art against all-comers. The UFC was a pay-per-view extravaganza that pitted all varieties of martial arts against each other in the first modern fighting competition without rules, judges, or time limits. The repeated victories of the Gracie Jiu-Jitsu practitioner against larger, stronger, and highly skilled fighters sparked a revolution in the martial arts world that has continued to this day. Today, everyone accepts that Gracie Jiu-Jitsu is the only martial art that enables you to survive the attack of a bigger, stronger assailant. I had achieved my objective.

Now, I have an even greater task – to expand the concept of self-defense beyond physical combat to include lifestyle changes that will enable you to defeat your internal assailants. That's self-defense in the fullest meaning of the term. Millions of Americans struggle with the related challenges of diet, weight control, and fitness. We hear that the United States is the most obese nation in history, that childhood obesity is epidemic, and that poor nutrition is increasing the rates of heart disease, diabetes, and cancer. In the face of these alarming trends, many people simply surrender just as they would if facing an attacker twice their size. In much the same way that Gracie Jiu-Jitsu revolutionized thinking about physical combat, I believe the Gracie Diet will revolutionize your thinking about healthy eating habits and help you win the fight against internal assailants such as: obesity, disease, and frailty. I promise you – you can do it!

Reading this book is the first step toward leading a healthier, more energetic life. In the pages that follow you'll find very specific, highly practical guidelines for optimizing your eating habits, controlling your weight, and maintaining that control for the rest of your life. In fact, as time passes, you'll find the routine becomes easier. As in jiu-jitsu, it's just a matter of consistently using the tools and techniques you've learned. But before you can start using those techniques, there are a few key principles you must understand.

First and foremost, you must embrace the basic metaphor of this book: Weight control is a matter of defending yourself in a fight against a ruthless opponent who will use every trick in the book to harm you. Of course, we both know that there really is no external enemy. The person who is eating unhealthy foods is the same person who's suffering the consequences. That's you. But for reasons that will become clear as we move ahead, it's important to start separating your negative, self-destructive impulses from the authentic "you" who wants a healthy and fulfilling life. This is really important, so let's look closely at exactly what it means.

Imagine that you're waiting in the checkout line of a supermarket – a perfect location to get mugged by unhealthy eating, just like a dark alley at midnight is a good place to get mugged by a thief. You've been walking the aisles looking at food for an hour or more. You're hungry – and maybe a little tired after a long day at work. So many choices and it's all so tasty! If you're like most people, some of your choices (maybe most of them) won't be the healthiest ones. So what? Why not? Don't you deserve a little enjoyment in life? So, you load up the soft drinks, snacks, comfort foods, and you're ready to go home.

But, you're not done yet – there's the checkout line. You're tired. You're tense. And, you're even hungrier now that you've been looking at food for hours. There's the annoying guy with a full shopping cart in front of you. There's the chattering cash register that's going to hit you up for plenty of money. There's the rack full of tabloids with one depressing story after another. You feel guilty for being interested in them, just like you feel guilty for some of the foods you've chosen. Why didn't you get in the other line? It's always so much faster. But wait. It's not all bad. There's a rack full of candy bars – just what you need to soothe your hunger and stress and to give you a quick energy boost…a life raft that will get you through this shipwreck of a checkout line. One of the candies really is a "Lifesaver!" So you grab a pack of Lifesavers® along with a Snickers® or an Almond Joy®. Life is good.

I think you get the picture. So now let's rewind the tape and play back the supermarket scenario from a self-defense perspective. When you entered the supermarket, you entered the arena of mortal combat – and your inner opponent was there waiting for you. That opponent has a thousand and one kicks, punches, and dirty tricks that he's ready and willing to use. Your opponent has a punch called, "What's the use?" He has a high kick called, "It's too late to change." He has an arm bar called, "Only a box of Oreo® cookies will stop the pain." These are powerful moves – and your opponent won't be satisfied if you simply surrender. Your opponent wants to kill you. The good news is that I have a counter for all of your opponent's attacks. In this book, I will show you how to defeat that opponent no matter how big and strong he is, or how many fights you've lost to him in the past.

Let's start by clarifying expectations about what you can achieve with this diet continuing with the self-defense metaphor. Some martial arts claim that they can enable anybody to overcome any adversary, no matter how dangerous or formidable, in very little time and without much training. This was the fantasy behind the ads that appeared in comic books fifty years ago. Who knows how many kids mailed away their allowances to learn the secret moves that could defeat all bullies. All they really got was a false sense of security and a serious misunderstanding of what effective self-defense training really involved. On the other end of the spectrum are those who refuse to believe that any amount of knowledge or training will enable them to survive an attack against a much larger, stronger adversary. At best, these skeptics acknowledge that the techniques might work in training, but don't believe they would work in a real fight.

Do either one of these viewpoints express your feelings about diet and weight control? Do you expect that this book will provide a quick fix – a silver bullet that will resolve your problems in the hour or so that's needed to read it from cover to cover? Or, do you simply dismiss it as yet another one of the hundreds, if not thousands, of fad diet books that will have come and gone over the years? Have you reached the point at which any diet advice is just too little, too late, or too difficult to bring about real change? Both of these extremes echo the voice of your opponent – and listening to either one of them will prevent you from achieving your dietary objectives.

Here are your first counterattacks. First, give yourself time. It's unlikely that you became overweight or underweight overnight. These conditions usually develop over months or years of poor eating habits. It will take time to reverse the conditions. The Gracie Diet will resolve the problems – but it will take more than a day or a week. Just as you can't instantly defend yourself against a strong-arm robber who is twice your size, you won't defeat this opponent in the time it takes to read the book. Success, in both situations, requires patience and discipline.

The Gracie Diet is not a quick weight-loss program. It is not a fad diet or even a restrictive one. In fact, it should not even be called a "diet" since it does not prohibit eating anything. The Gracie Diet is about education and reprogramming your eating habits. As you restructure your eating habits, a healthy diet will naturally become part of your way of life, as it has been for three generations of the Gracie family.

My uncle, Carlos Gracie, developed the Gracie Diet based on his observations of the effects of various food combinations. His original purpose was to ensure that all family members were ready to uphold the Gracie name in an unarmed fight with anyone, anywhere, and at any time. Uncle Carlos was not a doctor. He was a self-taught nutritionist who studied the writings of health experts. From these writings, he drew his own conclusions about the principles of healthy eating. Using himself and the rest of the Gracie family as participants in an experiment that lasted more than 65 years, he was able to fine tune and validate his conclusions.

I want to be very clear about the fact that, like my uncle, I am neither a medical doctor nor a credentialed nutritionist. The Gracie Diet has yet to be proven in science labs and test tubes. But, my health, my family members' health, and the health of thousands of our students testify to its benefits. For over 65 years, the dinner table has been our science lab, and the longevity and good health of those who have followed the Gracie Diet is all the evidence I need to know that it works. Fad diets come and go. Every year we see some new program promise to solve weight problems, lower cholesterol, improve heart function, slow aging, and on and on. Some of the diets produce short-term results but none of them stand the test of time. As a result, none of these diets can document long-term benefits. I know of no other regimen except the Gracie Diet that can point to more than 65 years of real life testing.

When I was growing up, I was often told that following the Gracie Diet would pay off after I turned 50. I'm now 58 years old. I base my certainty in the principles of our diet on some simple facts. I am free from most of the health problems that plague many people my age. I'm still able to do the same physical activities that I did thirty years ago. I can even keep up with my ten children...and the two-year-old only stops when he's sleeping!

In the 1930s when Uncle Carlos was in the early stages of his research, he pioneered the "self-defense" approach to health issues. He looked at people suffering from different complaints as if they were jiu-jitsu students and characterized their health problems as challenging opponents. My mother, for example, had suffered from serious gastro-intestinal problems early in her life. She was healed by a healthier way of eating and became a firm believer in the Gracie Diet. Gradually, my Uncle Carlos began building an almost magical reputation for helping people by modifying their eating habits.

I grew up watching Uncle Carlos and my father live long and healthy lives. They knew this was made possible by the Gracie Diet, and before I knew it the Diet became a way of life for me as well. I learned to prioritize the importance of what I ate because I knew each meal had a direct impact on my health. In the pages that follow, I'll teach you the strategies and tactics that I've embraced. I'll be "in your corner" at every meal. Just as I've taught chokes and arm locks to defeat any adversary, I'll train you in "dietary self-defense."

You'll learn to avoid certain combinations of foods – even some that give you pleasure – because you know they're not good for you. You'll learn the effect that self-discipline – or the lack thereof – will have on your life and on the lives of your loved ones. Although the reputation of our family is a result of our sensational accomplishments in the ring, our Diet made this possible by maximizing the potential of the Gracie warriors. Truly, the Gracie Diet has been our secret weapon. Now it's your turn to learn the secrets.

R.G.

PART ONE:

The Gracie Diet

CHAPTER 1:

Your Diet IS Your Life

Origins of the Gracie Diet

In 1914, a Japanese jiu-jitsu champion named Mitsuyo Maeda immigrated to Brazil. There, he met my grandfather, Gastão Gracie, a Brazilian scholar and businessman. Gastão helped Maeda settle in the new country, and in return Maeda taught jiu-jitsu to Carlos, my grandfather's oldest son. When the family moved to Rio de Janeiro in the early 1920s, Carlos, still in his teens, decided to teach jiu-jitsu. In order to promote his school, he issued open challenges to anyone who wanted a match. Over time, Carlos introduced his brothers to jiu-jitsu and they too became totally dedicated to the art. So, in 1925, they opened the first Gracie Jiu-Jitsu Academy.

My father, Helio Gracie, was the youngest of Carlos Gracie's brothers. When he was sixteen years old and physically rather frail, Helio began experimenting with different ways to apply the traditional Japanese techniques. By focusing on leverage, timing, and natural body movements, he found that he could increase the effectiveness of many of the techniques and make them work against much bigger and stronger opponents. Helio dissected and tested every move until he discovered how to make it work against virtually any opponent – he literally reinvented the Japanese martial art. Soon, he too was challenging all kinds of opponents to fight anytime and anywhere. Helio's unexpected victories catapulted him to stardom; he became the first sports legend in Brazilian history and came to be known as the father of Brazilian jiu-jitsu.

It was only when his brothers started demonstrating their abilities on the mat that Carlos, then in his late 20s, shifted his focus and found his true calling in life. He immersed himself in a variety of subjects related to body, mind, and spirit. His studies in philosophy, religion, and health established him as the spiritual leader of the Gracie family.

Since none of the Gracie brothers were physically gifted, they had to stay healthy in order to sustain the open challenge that had become the family hallmark. Optimal health was essential. This is what motivated Carlos to study the links between diet and physical performance. He began his research by reading a wide range of opinions from various health experts and nutritionists. Then, he narrowed his interest to food combining, which he saw as the most important aspect of nutrition. Eventually, he also studied the use of medicinal herbs.

I based this book on the diet principles that my Uncle Carlos discovered and that my family has followed for many years. I supplemented those principles with my own experience as an athlete, a parent, and a teacher. I'm certainly aware of the great number and variety of diet books on the market covering nearly every approach to eating. In fact, if someone were to publish a book suggesting that we shouldn't change anything in our eating habits, it might be a bestseller! But, I'm confident this book is like no other.

Your Diet Determines the Quality of Your Life

Simply put, your diet determines the quality of your life. It determines not just how you feel from day to day, but also how long you will live, how well you will live, and possibly how you will eventually die. It's common knowledge that unhealthy eating habits contribute to chronic illnesses or, at the very least, can result in obesity, malnutrition, or other imbalances that threaten your health. A poor diet can also seriously affect your mental and emotional health. The inability to participate in recreational activities can lead to isolation from friends and family, depression, and, of course, only accelerates the harmful effects of poor eating habits. I recall hearing an obese father lament, "My son wanted to throw the football but I couldn't get up off the couch." This situation is not only tough for the parent, but also affects the child.

Your eating habits begin to form at birth based on how and what your parents fed you. Essentially, your parents taught you how to eat. And your parents learned how to eat from their parents. I was fortunate to grow up in a family in which healthy eating was taken very seriously. My parents filled my baby bottles with papaya or figs blended with cheese or freshly squeezed watermelon juice blended with bananas and other natural foods. Today, my children's bottles contain the same fresh and nutritious foods – because that's what my parents taught me. I'm confident that my children will pass these good habits on to their children.

I realize that not everyone had the benefit of my role models and may have never developed good eating habits. I also know it's difficult to change habits ingrained in your life's routines since birth. But, your life depends on accepting the challenge to change and telling yourself, "That was then, this is now!" This commitment to change your diet and improve the quality of your life is perhaps the most wonderful gift you can give to yourself and your loved ones. You (and they) absolutely deserve it.

Dietary Decisions

We can learn much about natural eating habits by observing animals in the wild. Animals exhibit very specific eating habits that have evolved over thousands of years. They follow regular and simple diets that keep them healthy. Are there overweight giraffes or zebras? I don't think so. Nor do zebras need Tums®, Kaopectate®, or Metamucil® as long as they stick to their customary foods. Humans, on the other hand, face a more complicated situation. We not only have many more options than zebras or giraffes, but we were blessed with a uniquely powerful decision-making capability and, therefore, must contend with the internal opponent tempting us with unhealthy choices at every turn.

In a fight, an inexperienced person panics in the midst of what they perceive as total chaos. They act out of desperation and play right into the hands of a better-trained adversary. The unschooled fighter simply lacks the tools to win the fight. Their actions not only guarantee their defeat, but can even hasten that outcome. In a fight with a mugger, that can mean leaving yourself open to a punch or a choke. In a fight against the inner opponent, it means making food choices that will undermine your health and well-being. Imagine that your opponent sprinkled an invisible, tasteless poison on a container of ice cream. You would eat it without giving a thought to the deadly consequences. On the other hand, you wouldn't touch the ice cream if you knew of the poison. Just as in the fight against the mugger, your ability to recognize threats and respond with the proper counter will ensure your victory in the battle for your health when making dietary choices.

One of the least known dietary dangers is the negative impact that improper food combining has on your digestive system and overall health. Your inner opponent's most common and most successful tactic is to attack you through your taste buds. Most people simply follow their taste buds and mix foods without giving any thought to the implications of various food combinations. Put simply, taste drives our food selections and even determines the order in which we eat them. For example, many people want a sweet dessert after eating a typical American main course comprised of meat, vegetables, and starches. It just seems natural because that's how you ate as a child. The problem is that taste alone can drive us to combine foods that do not digest well together. The result is inefficient digestion as your body works harder to digest the food. The effects are real but often subtle, and soon they become part of everyday life. Poor food choices repeated every day, year after year, create an array of health issues. Without a disciplined dietary regimen, you're more likely to gain unnecessary weight and will have a difficult time shedding the extra pounds.

Learn to listen to your whole body, not just your taste buds. Your body tells you when it isn't operating at peak efficiency. The immediate stress of unhealthy eating may be just a subtle discomfort that varies from person to person. One person may feel a headache, another may have a stomachache, and a third may feel nothing at all. In this book, I'll show you how to recognize the signs of unhealthy food options. To me those signs are very clear, just as the mistakes of an untrained student are obvious when I'm teaching jiu-jitsu. Soon the mistakes will be obvious to you, too. And, so will the right choices. In time, you will find that the Gracie Diet, like Gracie Jiu-Jitsu, will produce maximum results from minimal effort. Specifically, the Diet enables the body to maximize the nutritional benefits of food while using minimal energy to digest it. Your body will function more efficiently and you will feel better as a result.

Is there medical or scientific proof that these combinations are healthy?

No. Although Carlos Gracie was not a doctor, he diligently studied the works of countless nutritionists, health professionals, and naturalists. These were the sources from which he drew his conclusions. Then, he used himself and the large number of family members as subjects for his research, which lasted more than 65 years. The final objective of any good diet is not only to increase longevity, but, more importantly, to ensure a good quality of life. Observing the long and healthy lives lived by brothers Carlos and Helio Gracie was enough to inspire me to follow in the same path. However, it is the life-changing impact that these eating habits have had on thousands of people, many of whom I have personally coached, that came to be the irrefutable evidence of the benefits of the Gracie Diet.

Points to Remember:

- You formed eating habits over many years, but you always have the power to change them. You can immediately begin to counter the negative effects of a bad diet by starting to eat properly today.

- Your body uses an incredible amount of energy to digest each meal. Any effort spent on maximizing the efficiency of the digestive process is effort well spent.

- Learning to manage the temptations elicited by your taste buds is the first step towards optimizing your health.

 THE GRACIE DIET IN A NUTSHELL

- *Only drink plain water or coconut water between meals.*
- *Wash your hands before every meal.*
- *Thoroughly wash all fruits and vegetables before consumption.*
- *Peel fruits before you eat them unless you are certain that the skin is free from pesticides.*

CHAPTER 2:

The Key to Good Health –
Proper Food Combinations

The Food Industry Isn't Interested in Your Health

Chefs all over the world strive to combine three elements in their meals: visual appeal, enticing aroma, and delicious taste. What about the health aspect of a meal? I have a friend who is a renowned chef in a high-end restaurant. When I asked him about this, he said, "Well, that's not a priority. Eating should be a pleasant experience, and I want to provide that for the guests in my restaurant. I always use the best ingredients." My friend's restaurant is indeed very successful. However, he is quite overweight, has health problems, and is on a strict diet that – for his own good – prevents him from eating the very foods he serves to others.

Sometimes even taste isn't a factor. I once met a young woman who won a prize from a national magazine for her original cake recipe. When she entered the contest, she learned that appearance rather than taste would determine the winner. The winning recipe had to look great on the pages of the magazine. After all, readers weren't going to eat the food; they were just going to look at it. So, she baked an amazingly colorful and beautifully shaped lemon cake. It happened to taste bland and was full of unhealthy ingredients, but those same ingredients enhanced the cake's structure and appearance. Her prize was a bicycle.

It gets worse. In a television commercial, breakfast cereal rains down into a bowl in slow motion. In the next shot, milk pours from the sky, followed by beautiful red strawberries that magically land perfectly spaced on the bed of cereal. Then, the cereal box descends to the left of the bowl accompanied by a full glass of orange juice. Wow! It's a perfect breakfast! The message is that any cereal that's so visually attractive probably tastes wonderful too. After all, anything that looks so good and tastes so good must be good for you as well. The emphasis is on visual appeal with the implication that it will also taste good. Some commercials will tout the health benefits of the food, but more often than not, as my friend the chef expressed it, the health benefit "is not really a priority."

If you grew up watching food commercials – and if nobody ever told you about the health consequences of eating food just because it looks wonderful – it's easy to understand why you would never stop eating it or stop feeding it to your children. It is not a coincidence that obesity is at an all-time high in the United States, the country with the most advertising dollars spent by the food industry. You might feel differently if you read the *Los Angeles Times* article (Maugh II, 2008) in which researchers found that "the arteries of many obese children and teenagers are as thick and stiff as those of 45-year-olds." It makes you wonder about the condition of their 45-year-old parents' arteries. That was not the topic of the article, but the implications are clear – just because a food looks good, doesn't mean that it's good for you.

Stories of the Healing Powers of the Gracie Diet

While Carlos was not a doctor, he was a keen observer and a self-taught nutritionist. He earned a reputation as a healer through his successes "curing" an array of health problems with his dietary guidance. His specialty was gastro-intestinal illnesses, and he often said, "No ulcer can resist me for thirty days!" Notably, he even treated the head physician at a renowned ulcer clinic in Rio de Janeiro. The doctor's ulcer was so bad that he scheduled himself for a surgical repair. Carlos convinced him to try the Gracie Diet during the weeks prior to the surgery. He taught the doctor's cook how to prepare healthy food combinations and directed the doctor to allow five hours between meals.

The doctor was skeptical. "What about my pain?" he said. "Everyone knows an ulcer patient needs to drink milk and eat as often as possible." But Uncle Carlos was firm: "Doctor, with all due respect, I am in charge now."

The doctor reluctantly agreed to follow the instructions and promised to report back in a few days. On the fourth day, he very excitedly reported that he had slept through the night for the first time in ages. By the tenth day, the pain was completely gone. By the end of the second week, the X-ray did not detect any traces of an ulcer. The doctor completed the 28-day program and became a believer in the Gracie Diet.

However, he told Carlos, "I cannot tell you how impressed I am. It's as if some kind of magic was performed before my very own eyes. I will be forever grateful to you. If there is ever anything you need, you can rest assured I will be there for you. The only thing I can never do is publicly admit that I was cured by someone who is not a doctor."

Carlos philosophically replied: "Doctor, I didn't treat you expecting publicity. I wanted to refine my treatment. It was in my best interest as well as yours."

On another occasion, a woman lost all of her teeth in a car crash. A renowned oral surgeon implanted new teeth, but the woman's body rejected the implants. The surgeon asked Carlos for his thoughts on a dietary program that would address the body's reaction to the surgery. Again, Carlos developed an eating regimen that worked when conventional medical procedures were at a loss.

You Have Nothing to Lose and Everything to Gain

Carlos believed that proper food combinations were the key to good health. He based this conclusion on hundreds of observations, although the aforementioned were two of the most dramatic. He also observed that improper food combinations were potentially harmful. You need not accept the full body of Carlos' work, but if you approach the Gracie Diet with an open mind, you'll find it much easier to follow in the early stages. After just two weeks, the results will speak for themselves and you'll need no more convincing. One of the first things you'll notice when eating the Gracie way is an increase in your energy level. You'll also find a decrease in the frequency of headaches, irregular bowel movements, heartburn, and stomachaches that can indicate a chronic health problem with unpredictable consequences. As your body becomes accustomed to healthy eating habits, you will be able to sense when something isn't right and will eventually be able to identify the cause of the problem.

I can't prove that the Gracie Diet is the best way to eat. I've been challenged on various aspects of the Diet over the years. The critics usually cite a lack of scientific evidence to support our claims or studies on nutrition and health that refute either the general concept of food combining, or more often, our observations on specific food combinations. Some have stated that the Gracie family's remarkable health is attributable to good genes more than good eating habits. Notably, no one has condemned the Diet in its entirety, and most acknowledged that, at worst, it will not harm you. I will say nothing to refute the naysayers other than to cite my own experiences and those of my very large family. The Gracie Diet has certainly withstood the test of time. For almost a century, the food combination concept has been the cornerstone of our lifestyle, providing abundant energy and outstanding health for a family that has become a symbol of efficiency in physical combat.

Interestingly, nutritionists are starting to champion many of the same ideas that my uncle had been promoting for decades. I find this to be a refreshing vindication and evidence that Carlos was indeed far ahead of his time. Once, more than 35 years ago in Brazil, he and I saw an Alka-Seltzer® commercial that proclaimed: "Eat anything you want! If you have indigestion, take an Alka-Seltzer and you'll feel great!" Carlos responded, "How ridiculous! They encourage you to eat wrong so that they can sell you the illusion of a cure. Why not promote healthy eating instead?" Then he added: "Like fish, most people die through their mouths!"

The human body naturally functions in perfect balance. Don't complicate things by feeding it the wrong foods! Eating right is easy. All you need is common sense and a willingness to learn some basic concepts. The purpose of this book is to teach you how to choose your foods and improve your eating habits. Do not be surprised if you find out that you can still eat many of the same foods you now enjoy, as long as you consider what you eat them with. Expect immediate improvements in your overall health!

It's Not What You Eat, It's What You Eat It With

While it's always best to eat high-quality organic foods, it's even more important that you properly combine your foods in each meal. A well-combined meal is not a matter of appearance, aroma, or even taste. Instead, the Diet combines foods to help prevent fermentation and blood acidity during the digestive process. When we say that certain foods "combine," we mean that mixing those foods in a meal is good for your weight and overall health. Foods that "do not combine," are those mixtures that inhibit digestion and, as a result, can undermine attempts to regulate your weight control and negatively affect your general well-being. In fact, proper food combination is at the core of the Gracie Diet.

The Gracie family's experience with the positive results of a diet focused on proper food combination is quite amazing. Furthermore, the impressive results achieved by non-family members validate the Diet.

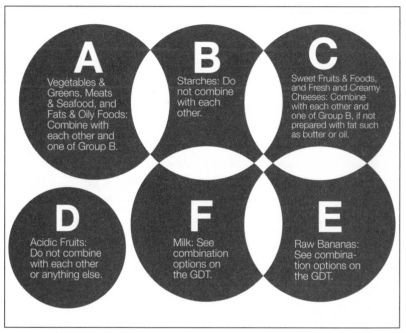

A Vegetables & Greens, Meats & Seafood, and Fats & Oily Foods: Combine with each other and one of Group B.

B Starches: Do not combine with each other.

C Sweet Fruits & Foods, and Fresh and Creamy Cheeses: Combine with each other and one of Group B, if not prepared with fat such as butter or oil.

D Acidic Fruits: Do not combine with each other or anything else.

F Milk: See combination options on the GDT.

E Raw Bananas: See combination options on the GDT.

Note: *Each intersection in the diagram above represents one properly combined meal possibility. For the complete list of foods and the combination guidelines that govern each group, please reference the Gracie Diet Table on pages 51-53.*

Will I have to give up my favorite foods to follow the Diet?
A friend told me that after following the Gracie Diet for a few weeks he was feeling great. Then he decided to go out to dinner and ordered his old favorite dish. The next morning he told me, "My favorite dish made me feel sick all night. I never want to eat it again!" The secret to good health is to learn to like the things that are good for you. Next time you decide you can't resist eating a certain dish, remind yourself that your meals shouldn't be determined by taste alone. Make the wise choice! However, if the ingredients of your favorite dish don't combine according to the Gracie Diet, often, the dish can be modified to do so. Besides, who is to say that you can't adopt a new favorite dish?

Points to Remember:

- The Gracie Diet is largely based on the fact that eating foods in proper combinations will benefit your health.

- Even if foods taste good, they can still be harmful if not eaten with compatible foods. The key is to learn to like what is good for you.

- Try the Gracie Diet for two weeks – the changes you see and feel will convince you to stay the course for the rest of your life.

 THE GRACIE DIET IN A NUTSHELL

- *For juicing apples, melons, pineapples, carrots, etc., use a juicer.*
- *When juicing watermelon or grapes use a blender. After blending the fruit, strain the mixture through a Gracie Juice Bag into a bowl. (Get your Gracie Juice Bag at www.GracieDiet.com)*
- *For the ultimate frozen treat use the Champion Juicer to make ice cream from frozen fruits and fruit blends.*
- *Prepare the juice only at mealtime. The nutritional value of freshly squeezed juice diminishes almost instantly if you let it sit.*

CHAPTER 3:

Where Are You Now?

Food is Everywhere!

The availability of food has always determined our diets. Once driven by our ability to hunt, gather, or cultivate, today our food choices are seemingly limitless with nothing to shape our eating habits other than personal preferences and cultural influences. Some people use food as a stress reliever – snacking on chips or drinking a soda much like a bottle calms a baby. Others follow highly restrictive "health food" diets seeking peace of mind in knowing that they are avoiding pesticides, additives, cholesterol, carcinogens, and other perceived dangers. In both cases, the experience of eating becomes a form of treatment, like taking medicine. But whether someone is a fast-food addict or a health-food devotee, relatively few people are really aware of what motivates them to eat the way they do.

Establish a Base Point

In order to change, it helps to establish a base point to improve your understanding of your dietary habits. So, let's begin by assessing your current eating and drinking behaviors by evaluating your response to the following thirty questions. A brief discussion of the possible answers follows each question. You may read the discussion prior to answering the questions, but be honest with yourself. Your responses will provide a dietary snapshot of what you eat, when you eat, and how you eat. The results may surprise you as most people take this fundamental life behavior for granted based on years of eating habits handed down by parents and shaped by daily routines. If you're not satisfied with your diet and how it makes you feel based on your responses to the questions, then I suggest you give the Gracie Diet a try. You really have nothing to lose as the regimen is easy to follow and you will still be able to eat most of your favorite foods. Reassess your eating habits after you've been following the Diet for a few weeks. You may find your answers have changed as much as your eating habits. Feel free to write your answers in the book, or on a separate sheet of paper.

1. What are your goals for the Gracie Diet?

The way human beings think about what they eat has changed considerably in the last hundred years. Diets consisting of meat, potatoes, and dairy products once defined a healthy meal. We even found virtue in being overweight as it signified the ability to eat well and often. Large physical size also conveyed an image of power and importance. Many of America's wealthiest businessmen were overweight or obese. William Howard Taft, President of the United States from 1909-1913 and later a Justice of the Supreme Court, weighed more than 300 pounds and sometimes needed help getting out of the bathtub. In contrast, we viewed very thin people as poor, weak, and even sickly. Today, we know that excessive fat is unhealthy and it's no longer fashionable. Not surprisingly, the positive views once associated with plumpness are now reserved for thin people. We associate being overweight not only with being unattractive and unhealthy, but also with being poor. In fact, most of America's obese people reside in the nation's poorest regions. Despite the changed attitudes toward excessive weight and the health risks associated with high-fat diets, Americans are still among the world's most obese people.

It's difficult to accept that anyone would work at being unhealthy and physically unattractive. Yet, these are the conditions commonly associated with poor eating habits. On the other hand, you may be satisfied with your current weight and appearance, but what does the inside of your body look like? Your goals may pertain more to how you feel, rather than how you look. If you're not comfortable with how you look, or how you feel, then do something about it. Making radical changes in your diet won't happen by itself. It will take consistent effort, especially at the beginning. So you'll need worthwhile goals in order to sustain your motivation. Do you have those goals? What are they?

2. What lifestyle changes will your goals require? Are you prepared to make those changes?

The Gracie Diet is more than just a list of foods and how to prepare them. The Diet is really a way of life. Following the Diet means making some real changes – not just in what you eat, but in your whole orientation toward food. And since food is such a basic part of what we do every day, changing your thinking about food really means changing your thinking about your life in general. I can say with total confidence that the changes will be positive ones, but change of any kind doesn't always come easily, especially if you're not well prepared for it.

For example, throughout this book I'll be emphasizing the fact that in order to follow the Gracie Diet, you can no longer decide what to eat simply on the basis of taste. For most people, this is a big change. It means ignoring all those advertisements for fast food hamburgers that have been carefully crafted by expert marketers. It means avoiding the most "taste tempting" items on a restaurant menu, or maybe even avoiding the restaurant itself. Please note, this does not mean you will no longer be able to enjoy delicious meals, you can indeed create delightful food combinations that agree with the Gracie Diet, but you will no longer allow taste to dominate/manipulate your choices in food. In general terms, the Gracie Diet asks you to forego a certain level of instant gratification from your food in favor of continued well-being. As you begin to change your eating habits, just be aware you're making that choice. As time goes on, you'll know it was the right one.

3. How high is your motivation for reaching your goals?

Success depends on approaching the Diet with a strong sense of motivation that you can sustain over a long period of time. It's normal to start something new with great enthusiasm and excitement. The initial "high" associated with new and different activities frequently fades over time as we hit plateaus in our progress or find the undertaking to be more difficult than expected. Successful progress in both the Diet and Gracie Jiu-Jitsu relies on having a strong foundation based in part on immediate, sustained positive feedback and on the knowledge that you will win in the long run. Many times a match will seem to be going against us, but the whole orientation of Gracie Jiu-Jitsu is toward winning in the end, no matter how long it takes. This is why I have been opposed to time limits in sanctioned fights. Gracie Jiu-Jitsu competitors are motivated for the long haul. There's no time limit for real-life challenges, so there shouldn't be time limits in the most lifelike form of martial arts. Be aware of the difference between excitement and motivation. The main difference is sustainability. Excitement comes and goes – and it always goes eventually. Motivation means "whatever it takes," for an hour, a day, or a lifetime.

4. Who will support you in following the Diet?

Breaking old habits and forming new ones is difficult. The support of family and friends can help with the transition. Changing eating habits is especially difficult because often your routine is tied to factors beyond your direct control – like family schedules. It's likely that your family has eating habits formed over many years, if not several generations.

When a family member suddenly decides to change the routine in any way, it's natural for some or all to resist the initiative. But, if your family and friends are not fully supportive and willing to compromise their own routines for your sake, then your challenge will be more difficult.

The best way to enlist support is to emphasize the positive health benefits of the Diet. After all, the resistance has more to do with disrupting comfortable routines than with your healthy objectives. If you can convince them that the change is not only good for you, but also for your family and friends, then it's more likely that they will support you. There's also a good chance that the benefits of healthy eating will be so obvious that everyone will want in on your newfound energy. This has been a way of life in the Gracie family for three generations. What's worked so well in our family can also work in yours.

5. What is most difficult for you in managing your weight?

For many people, two erroneous beliefs are at the heart of their inability to manage body weight. The first fallacy is that you can't control your weight…that you just can't win because it's all too complex, powerful, and overwhelming. This is something we also see in beginning jiu-jitsu students. If faced with an opponent who's bigger and stronger, they're convinced they're going to get beat up even before anything happens. They don't understand that the whole point of jiu-jitsu is to empower the weak against the strong, based on information, efficiency, and confidence. So the initial principle a student needs to grasp is trust in the system. Trust that it really is possible to defend against a seemingly formidable adversary. And remember: That adversary is not chocolate or fried chicken or mashed potatoes. The real opponent is the enemy within – your belief that you can't change and you can't achieve your goals. So, you've got to defend yourself from yourself by developing confidence in the Diet.

The second misconception is that you're more tired than you actually are. This mindset holds people back at the very moment when real progress is just becoming possible. It sets in when you hit the inevitable plateau where the novelty of a new behavior is gone and fruits of the labor have yet to appear. Prepare for this by knowing that the high of beginning a new lifestyle is a delightful, but short-term feeling. One morning you're going to wake up and say, "Keeping track of these food groups is too much trouble," or, "I'm not losing weight fast enough." If you're expecting the plateau, you'll be better prepared to remain committed to the regimen and achieve your goals. If you succumb to the letdown and quit the Diet, you will have allowed the enemy within to defeat you.

6. What can you do to make following the Diet easy and enjoyable?

You're already taking the first step by answering these questions and establishing a base point from which to start. Record your answers so that when you reassess your progress in a few weeks, you will appreciate the changes in your eating habits. Of course, you will already feel the difference, but seeing your progress on paper helps you to really appreciate your accomplishment.

7. What was your body weight at each of the following ages?
- 15/20   - 20/30   - 30/40   - 40/present

8. What do you believe would be your ideal weight at this time?

9. Have you followed any other diets for an extended period of time?

10. How long did you stick with the diets?

11. What were your results?

12. What were the positives and negatives of the diets you followed?

13. Why did you stop?

14. What did you learn from these programs regarding your weight?

15. Why do you want to begin the Gracie Diet now?

16. Which meals do you regularly eat?
- Breakfast
- Brunch
- Lunch
- Dinner

17. When do you snack?
- Morning
- Afternoon
- Evening
- Late at night
- Throughout the day

18. What are your favorite snack foods?

19. How often do you eat in restaurants or order food delivered?

20. How many times each day do you eat the following foods?
- Starch (bread, cereal, pasta, rice, potato)
- Fruits
- Vegetables
- Dairy (milk, yogurt)
- Meat, fish, poultry
- Fat (butter, margarine, mayonnaise, oil, salad dressing)
- Sweets (candy, cake, regular soda, juice)

21. How much of these beverages do you drink daily?
- Water
- Coffee
- Tea
- Soda
- Juice
- Alcohol

22. What are the most difficult times of the day for you to stay within a diet?
- Morning
- Afternoon
- Early Evening
- Late Evening
- All Day

23. What do you see as your major food temptations?
- Sweets – candy, cookies, cakes, sodas
- Starches – breads, potatoes, pasta, chips
- Butter
- Meats

24. During holidays or when eating in a restaurant, do you:
- Eat whatever you want to enjoy?
- Eat whatever you want and then eat more carefully for the next few days?
- Stick with your diet plan in these situations?

25. How frequently do you eat in each of these environments?
- While working, at your desk, or elsewhere
- With friends and/or family
- Alone
- In front of the television

26. How often are your meals:
- Home cooked
- Fast food
- A mix of fast food and home cooked
- Only healthy foods
- Restaurant / take out or delivery

27. Pick your favorite part of a restaurant meal:
- Bread / Chips
- Appetizers
- Salad
- Main Course
- Dessert

28. How often do you take second portions?
- Never
- Occasionally
- Almost always

29. How often do you eat meat?
- Never
- Occasionally
- Quite often

30. When you prepare or shop for food, what is most important?
- Your health
- Your family's health
- How the food will taste
- What will fit your budget

Now that you have a base point for your current eating habits, you're ready to take action. In the next chapter, we'll discuss the hardest part of the Diet – forming healthy eating habits.

Having the Willpower to Resist Temptation... And Feel Good About It Afterwards

Following the Diet has positive benefits beyond improving your health. Surprising as it may seem, the sense of responsibility and personal discipline that I've found in following the Gracie Diet have been the real foundation of my training in jiu-jitsu, not the other way around. My ability to resist social pressures and to do the right thing for my health has set an example for my family and friends with far-reaching, long-lasting effects. Through the Gracie Diet, you will learn to conquer yourself, and once you do that, nothing is impossible.

Points to Remember:

- The Gracie Diet is more than just a list of food combinations. It's the beginning of a new and healthier way of life.

- Your motivation for a healthy transformation is much more important than any aspect of your current physical condition.

- Never let yourself feel that change is beyond your control. You have the power to defeat any internal adversary, starting today!

 THE GRACIE DIET IN A NUTSHELL

- *Stay away from canned or bottled fruit juices, even if it says that they are 100% natural and have no preservatives.*
- *When eating sweet fruits (Group C), you don't have to eat cheeses (Group C) and a starch (Group B) with your meal, especially if you want to lose weight.*
- *The fiber in some fruits will quickly fill your stomach. If you opt to juicing instead, you'll increase the nutritional value of the meal.*
- *Keep a stock of your favorite fruits and vegetables. Plan ahead so that when it's time to eat, you'll have everything you'll need.*

CHAPTER 4:

The Hard Part –
Changing Your Eating Habits

Make Healthy Eating a Habit

Your health should be the most important thing in the world to you. In the Gracie family, we take our health very seriously and believe that refueling your body with food is perhaps the single most important part of your daily routine. A meal at our house is almost ceremonial. It starts with the food selection. As a boy in Brazil, I watched Uncle Carlos and my father buy fruits at the central produce market every week. They fussed over every selection to ensure that we not only had the right foods, but also that they were fresh, ripe, and tasty so that the children would enjoy the meals and grow to love the Diet. It paid off big time for me! Once a week at dawn for the last thirty years, I've gone to the wholesale central produce market in downtown Los Angeles come rain or shine to buy crates of fruits for the family. This is a habit handed down to me by my father that I have made a weekly ritual.

The ability to break and form habits is really at the heart of any regimen. The more you take control of your eating habits, the more you will find that you can take control of all other aspects of your life. When you can say "no" to your favorite dish because you have learned it contains foods that do not combine with each other; or when you can say to yourself: "I'm hungry and want to eat something, but it isn't time yet," and you make the conscious decision to drink a glass of water instead, and realize that you didn't die of starvation; or better yet, when you sit down to enjoy your favorite meal, and you decide to fill yourself to 80% instead of 110% because you are beginning to understand that the purpose of eating is the nourishment of our bodies not the stuffing of our faces, you will be surprised by the increased power you will have to make important decisions, especially when you are away from the dinner table.

This re-education process is like learning a new skill – like sewing, playing the piano, bowling, or flying a helicopter. You must follow a plan, which includes getting quality instruction, buying the necessary equipment, and committing time to it. It doesn't matter how much time goes by, if we have fond memories of a fun and positive hobby or activity from our past, the thought of it will always bring us joy. Many times these very activities serve as motivators as we age. So stick with the Diet – it could become the most pleasant and rewarding experience of your life.

Changing Habits Requires a Plan

During the thirty years I've been working with people to change their eating habits, I've learned one very important fact: If the plan fails, it's usually because people fail to plan. Make the time to study and understand the Diet, so that you are less likely to get confused, make mistakes, get frustrated, and give up. Otherwise, you may become discouraged, revert to old eating habits, and accept the physical and psychological consequences of a lost battle. That won't help your self-esteem. Often, you don't feel the chains of habit until they are too strong to break. Basic behaviors just don't change by themselves.

I've found the key to forming new habits is to start with small changes. For example, try to brush your teeth with your weak hand for seven days. At first, you find yourself forgetting to make the change because your brushing habits have become such a deeply ingrained reflex. Store your toothbrush on the opposite side of the sink. This will influence your habit-forming awareness, and help create a framework for a new way of thinking about food.

Likewise, you can ease into the Gracie Diet by making simple changes to your eating habits. You'll quickly find that the Diet really isn't as radical as you may have originally thought and that the guidelines are not difficult to follow. For example, despite my personal preference not to eat meat, the Diet allows for meat consumption in combination with the right foods. Again, my objective is to show everyone that no matter what your current eating habits are, there is a way for you to improve them. Sometimes, all you need to do is to avoid one simple ingredient.

You have been eating a certain way all of your life and now you have decided to explore a different way. You really have nothing to lose and everything to gain. After all, if you don't like this new way, you can always go back to your old eating habits. However, I am certain that the noticeable difference in how you feel will motivate you to make better choices and that will result in a positive cycle of endless possibilities.

Current Weekly Food Routine

Let's further develop your current base point by taking your "diet pulse." The first step is to use the following chart to record everything you eat for one week. Document every detail, including meal times, types of salad dressings, drinks, snacks, desserts, bread types, and how full you feel after the meal. In fact, use the vertical column as a "gas tank gauge" and treat each box as 20% of your "tank." Be sure to record your starting weight as well. Feel free to write your answers in the book, or on a separate sheet of paper.

List Your Current Eating Habits

	BREAKFAST	SNACK	LUNCH
MON	TIME:	TIME:	TIME:
TUE	TIME:	TIME:	TIME:
WED	TIME:	TIME:	TIME:
THUR	TIME:	TIME:	TIME:
FRI	TIME:	TIME:	TIME:
SAT	TIME:	TIME:	TIME:
SUN	TIME:	TIME:	TIME:

Be As Detailed As Possible

SNACK	DINNER	SNACK
TIME:	TIME:	TIME:
TIME:	TIME:	TIME:
TIME:	TIME:	TIME:
TIME:	TIME:	TIME:
TIME:	TIME:	TIME:
TIME:	TIME:	TIME:
TIME:	TIME:	TIME:

Doesn't it take a lot of time and work to prepare these meals?
For breakfast, at least three or four days a week, I prepare a smoothie made from bananas blended with a freshly squeezed fruit juice of watermelon, cantaloupe, or red delicious apples, plus a teaspoon of cream cheese. Peeling five bananas and putting them in the blender takes less than one minute. The process of washing, cutting, and juicing a cantaloupe can also be done in less than five minutes (We use the Champion Juicer – www.GracieDiet.com). Blending the ingredients takes less than one minute, and the clean-up takes about five minutes. So, there you have it – a delicious and healthy breakfast prepared in about 12 minutes. I guarantee that you will feel a lot better than if you had a bowl of cereal with milk, a glass of grapefruit juice, and a cup of coffee.

Points to Remember:

- Small changes are the easiest to make. Don't feel that you have to change all your eating habits immediately.

- The discipline you develop by taking control of your dietary habits will lead to success in all areas of your life.

- The Gracie Diet as a whole has proven itself over many years. It won't fail you, as long as you don't fail it.

 THE GRACIE DIET IN A NUTSHELL

- *When eating cooked foods (Group A), treat yourself to raw nuts such as cashews, walnuts, Brazil nuts, and almonds for additional protein.*

- *Most people prefer toasted and salted nuts, but try to eat the raw versions. Start by mixing some raw nuts with toasted nuts and gradually wean yourself off of the processed variety.*

- *Salads are great, but to get the most out of your vegetables try juicing them. Start with plain carrot juice and then try mixing it up with other veggies, see Group A.*

- *Vegetable juice (Group A) goes particularly well with an avocado sandwich.*

CHAPTER 5:

Getting Started

The beauty of the Gracie Diet is that you can eat almost anything. The key to good health is to learn how to combine your favorite foods with compatible foods to ensure efficient digestion and maximize the nutritional benefits. After all, a watermelon is a watermelon! What I am suggesting is that you learn to eat it with toast and cheese instead of eating it with chicken and pasta. I expect you to have questions regarding this new way of eating. Let me assure you that in the pages that follow, not only will you find the answers to your questions but also new outlooks on eating that will inspire you to reinvent yourself! The best way to appreciate how easy it is to follow the Diet, is to try it.

Three Steps to a Newer, Healthier, and Happier You

Most diets fail because they require too much change too quickly. In order to simplify your transition onto the Gracie Diet, we have developed the following three phase integration plan that will gradually introduce the Gracie Diet into your life. To ensure a smooth transition, you will spend one week on each phase before moving on to the next. At each phase you will introduce a new Gracie Diet principle that you will adhere to in addition to those from the preceding weeks. Don't stress over the process. Remember, it took many years for you to develop your current habits and you can't change them overnight. Imagine if suddenly you had to use your weak hand to do everything. Simple tasks such as moving the mouse on your computer, brushing your teeth, or dialing on a telephone would be very difficult – at first. Changing your eating habits is very similar, only harder. If you stray from the path on occasion, no worries... just get back on it as soon as you can. Use some of the age-old memory joggers to help you stay on task – tie a string to your watch or place a sticker on your computer screen or on the dashboard of your car. Do whatever it takes, but take that first step!

Phase 1:
Space your meals at least 4 ½ hours apart.

There is a theory that supports the idea of consuming several small meals throughout the day, based on the fact that the digestive process always working will cause the body to constantly "burn calories." However, according to the Gracie Diet, this is not recommended. Although the digestive process will indeed consume a lot of energy, there is one major factor that must be considered in this equation, which is: The chemical reactions resulting from the continuous addition of foods before the digestion is completed, will increase fermentation and blood acidity. You must space your meals at least 4 ½ hours apart (4 hours for children) to allow for the complete digestion of a meal. This is non-negotiable! Your body works to digest food. You allow your body to rest in between meals by completely digesting one meal before starting another. On the other hand, you overwork and exhaust your body when it's constantly digesting food. You only need three meals a day. Give up the snacks and limit yourself to water in between meals. I guarantee you will not starve. Once you have successfully spaced your meals for a period of one week, move on to Phase 2.

Phase 2:
Eliminate desserts and sodas.

Most of us crave sweets. The Diet allows you to eat sweets. In fact, you can eat as much as you'd like. The challenge is to learn how and when to eat them. The objective of this phase is to wean you off of unhealthy sweets that combine fat (oil, butter, etc.) with sugar. If, after your main meal, you are still hungry, it's better to eat more of the same than to complicate digestion by adding an incompatible sweet to the mix. Once you complete Phase 3, we'll introduce many delicious options that will quell your hunger for sweets. Believe me, I have a sweet tooth. But, I'm able to completely satisfy my craving by making a full meal of sweets such as fruits, honey, dates, fresh cheeses, etc. In the meantime, if you want to eat fruit, you can have it as one of the three meals of the day, but not as dessert or a snack anymore. If you miss the carbonation of sodas, switch to sparkling water. Once you have spent one week spacing your meals and avoiding unnecessary sweets, you're ready for Phase 3.

Phase 3:
Do not mix different starches within the same meal.

Eat only one starch per meal. Instead of a hamburger (that comes with two or more buns) and fries (wheat and potatoes), have two hamburgers and no fries or the meat patties (without the buns) and all the fries you want. Be especially attentive when you go to a restaurant and they drop the complimentary breadbasket on your table. If you want to eat that bread (wheat) while they prepare your food, then you should avoid anything that is derived from another starch. Instead, you will have to order something that is made with the same starch (wheat) i.e. pasta, pizza, hamburger, a wheat tortilla, etc. Everyone in Brazil grew up eating rice and beans. We never had it at the Gracie household. People often argued that due to the restrictions of the Diet we were missing out on one of the greatest pleasures of life. My father would often make me open my mouth to show off my cavity-free teeth. I always believed that I helped him win the argument.

Once you've integrated these three fundamental habits into your eating routine, you will appreciate the Diet's simplicity and, more important, you will begin to feel the positive effects of healthy eating. In Chapter 7, I will introduce you to the Gracie Diet food groups and teach you how to combine your foods, and then I will provide you with a 14-day meal plan that you can use to strategize your meals until you become comfortable with all the combination guidelines, but for now, let's focus on your first meal.

Your First Meal on the Gracie Diet

Your first meal should be a well-planned positive experience that inspires you to repeat it. I recommend you try a Gracie Diet fruit-based (Group C) meal. Try sharing this meal with a friend or a loved one. If you have children, I recommend that you bring them in for this because it's a great opportunity to plant a seed in their heads. Let them experience a sweet meal that is natural and healthier than candy bars and a soda. If they like the fruit meal, ask them if they would like to eat it once a week. There is a good chance they will like it and then it will be easier to try another meal. Educating someone on how to make healthy choices is the best present you can give them, especially your children. They will appreciate and respect you for that.

From this point on, you will take control, not only of your health through purpose and awareness of everything you eat, but, more importantly, you will practice a discipline that will increase your self-esteem and that will create endless possibilities! Eat to live, don't live to eat!

HERE ARE THREE SUGGESTIONS:

1) Pears, cottage cheese, and honey.

Selection: There are acidic and there are sweet pears. Make sure you use the sweet kind (D'anjou, Comice, etc.) They should look nice (no bruises), and will probably not be ripe, so you may have to wait a few days for them to be ready.

Preparation: Whenever they are ripe (soft to the touch), and it's mealtime, you should wash and peel them. Cut them into pieces, put them into a bowl with a spoon of cottage cheese and pour some honey over.

Serving: 2-3 pears per person.

Equipment: A peeler or a knife.

2) Dates and cream cheese with crackers and watermelon juice.

Selection: When in season, find a ripe watermelon, some crackers and cream cheese at your local supermarket and look for Madjool dates at your local health food store. Store the watermelon in the refrigerator the night before your meal.

Preparation: Place 6-8 dates onto a bowl with warm water for 60 seconds to loosen the skin. Then gently wash out the skin. With the tip of a knife, open the date and pick out the seed. Spread the cream cheese on the crackers and put the prepared dates on top. (Video tutorial available at *www.GracieDiet.com*)

Next, wash the watermelon, and slice enough to fill the blender halfway. Use a knife to chop into small enough pieces so that the blender blades will catch it. Do not add water, after blending for 15-20 seconds, pour it through a Gracie Juice Bag into a bowl, twist the opening to close the bag, and squeeze the juice out. (Video tutorial available at *www.GracieDiet.com*)

Serving: 1-2 people.

Equipment: A blender, a Gracie Juice Bag, a bowl, and a knife.

3) Apple juice, bananas, and cream cheese smoothie.

Selection: Use red apples and make sure the bananas are ripe.

Preparation: Wash and peel 4 red apples. Cut them into slices to fit the juicer. Pour the juice into a blender. Add 4-5 bananas and a teaspoon of cream cheese (optional) and blend it for 30-60 seconds. (Video tutorial available at *www.GracieDiet.com*)

Servings: 1-2 people.

Equipment: A juicer and a blender.

Aren't all these fresh fruits and vegetables very expensive?
I believe that money spent on natural foods today is money saved on medical bills tomorrow. You would be amazed at how much money you spend for snack foods, candy, or coffee with a pastry. Apply that money toward healthy foods and I think you'll find your food budget has increased very little, if at all. More important, you'll feel good all of the time – and that is priceless.

Points to Remember:

• Space your meals at least 4 ½ hours apart. Do not eat anything in between.

• Never eat dessert or drink sodas.

• Don't mix different starches within the same meal.

 THE GRACIE DIET IN A NUTSHELL

- *Avocado is a great substitute for meats and fish as it is protein-rich and toxin-free.*

- *Eat lots of dark, leafy greens.*

- *Choose fresh and mild cheeses such as cottage, ricotta, cream, Monterey Jack, etc., over the sharp, spicy, or aged ones like Roquefort and Camembert.*

- *When cheese is melted, it falls under Group A. When cheese is fresh, it falls under Group C.*

PART TWO:

Using the Gracie Diet

CHAPTER 6:

A Family Affair

Throughout this book, I've cited my childhood experiences as one of the most important factors in forming my own eating habits. The examples set by my relatives have stayed with me all of my life and I am now passing these habits to my children. Often, we only recognize and appreciate good habits once we're adults. Children almost always follow their hearts and their stomachs before they follow their heads... and both are organs without reasoning capabilities, so they don't always point in the right direction! My siblings and I were fortunate to not only have good examples set for us, but also to have parents who were so committed to our health that they trained us to eat properly by feeding us what was healthy and not allowing us to eat that which was not. The most powerful tool of all was their personal example. In fact, example isn't the best way to educate, it's the only way. With that in mind, I encourage you to eat well not only for your own health, but also to set an example for your children and put them on the road to good health.

The Power of Personal Example

The Gracie Diet is easy for me to follow because it's all I've ever known. There were no sodas, chocolate chip cookies, or candy bars to be found anywhere in the house...period. We ate when it was time to eat and if we got hungry before mealtime, a glass of water solved the problem. If not, we drank another one. No one ever starved to death. As a parent, I applied the same rules with my children and achieved the same positive results – children who, from birth, knew how and when to eat nutritious, healthy foods. I recognize your situation may be very different from mine.

I have heard many stories about the challenges families face when starting the Gracie way of eating. At first, everyone will be curious and want to try the meals – especially the fruit meals and smoothies. Their enthusiasm then quickly fades at the prospect of buying a juicer, keeping fresh fruit on hand, tracking food combinations, or modifying meal times. Don't let the waning interest dissuade you. Remember our discussion about the difficulty of breaking deeply ingrained habits and that you can't force a person to change their ways. They must decide on their own if the potential payoff is worth the sacrifice. The difficult part is accepting that you will be improving your health while your other family members will continue ruining theirs. The more aware you become, the more painful it is to ignore them.

The youngest ones should make the transition with ease (if you and your spouse work together). For the first six months, feed your infant nothing but breast milk. Usually infants will eat every three hours. Then, you should introduce mashed fruits like bananas or papaya once a day (make sure the fruits are ripe and sweet tasting). Soon thereafter, you can add a meal of mashed vegetables, soups, etc. to the daily routine. Avoid acidic (Group D) fruit meals for youngsters. As you introduce heavier foods, the child will naturally be able to wait a little longer in between meals. Eventually, the goal is to get the child on a comfortable routine of eating Gracie Diet compliant meals every four hours.

A Quick and Simple Way to Kick the Junk Food Habit

Kids only think about taste - because it provides instant gratification. They simply don't care about long-term, harmful consequences. When you cut out the junk food, you have to fill the "junk food void" with an explanation. Keep it simple and honest. Tell them that you are going to cut down the junk food because it is not good for them. Then, get all of it out of the house and never bring it back in! The key element for this to work is that there can't be any candy bars lying around, sodas in the refrigerator, or ice cream in the freezer. That means for everyone in the household. As you implement this new rule, expect a certain level of discontent from the troops. Do not feel sorry or get confused if you see tears or tantrums. Instead, take a deep breath and be fascinated by their dependency on junk food. Realize the seriousness of the situation and use it as a motivator to help you focus on your child's well-being. They will thank you later if they are kept out of the statistics on diabetes or the ever-growing number of obese children. Young children may have acquired a taste for "junk food" but at least they can't drive to the store. They will only have access to it if you bring it home. Don't do it anymore. If you know it is not good for them, why would you?

What to Do When Kids Demand Junk Food

You must be patient and understand that they may go through withdrawals, just like a drug addict. In order to deal with that, you may want to have some sugarless gum stashed away for an emergency. With the older kids, you will need a different strategy. It is not wise to force them into it. There is a risk of rebellion because they may not have the understanding of the healthy-versus-unhealthy mindset. Furthermore, they have access to everything at school or at the local store. The best approach is communication and patience. Remind them that the saying is "An apple a day..." not, "A Hershey bar a day..." – and that eating junk food will have negative consequences in the future.

The Ultimate Halloween Trick

Halloween is a fun holiday filled with cool costumes, cool social events, and lots of candy. In the Gracie household, we use it as an opportunity to teach discipline and willpower. When the kids come home with their bags full of goodies, we pour the contents on the carpet and we separate everything into categories based on the type of treat. We let the kids keep a few pieces of gum and maybe one or two lollipops, with the understanding that the rest is not good for them and must go into the trash. I praise the kids for being strong enough to collect so much candy and not eat it, and I remind them that their remarkable self-control will pay dividends in the long run.

How to Win the Kids Over, One Bite at a Time

Eating is near the top of the list of pleasures. As you learn to prepare your meals the Gracie way, I am sure you will win over other family members, one bite at a time! Always encourage everyone else to try it. Whenever my kids brought friends over, I made sure they tried a fruit meal from the Gracie Diet. They loved it – and I would use those opportunities to explain the general concept of the Diet to our guests, in order to teach my own children. The surprise and curiosity on the guests' faces reminded my kids that they were eating something out of the ordinary, something special. It raised their level of consciousness about healthy eating. Gradually, as my children learned the concepts, they grew comfortable enough to do the explaining themselves.

How to Inspire Your Loved Ones

If all of the above fails, then try for a partial conversion to the Diet. Consider, for example, reducing junk food consumption for one week to once every-other day instead of daily. Then, try to cut out junk food every-other two days for the second week, and so on. Maybe even say something like: "Let's see how much we save on candy bars and sodas for a month and use the money for a new video game, or a new outfit, instead."

What easy items can a parent prepare for their child's lunch?
Dates and cream cheese on pita or sourdough bread, or raisin bread and Monterey Jack cheese sandwich, with cantaloupe pieces and a bottle of water. Send it in a small lunch box with an ice pack. Alternate that with a couple of bananas and a red apple. In time, as they learn about the combinations it is OK for the kids to eat at the cafeteria. Remind them to stay away from the sauces. Be sure to talk with them and guide them on the process by explaining the importance and benefits of good health.

Points to Remember:

- Your motivation and success with the Gracie Diet will increase when you realize that you're not doing this for yourself alone.

- Achieving and sustaining good health will benefit everyone around you, especially members of your own family.

- The best way – and perhaps the only way – to help your children develop a healthy lifestyle is for you to lead by example.

 THE GRACIE DIET IN A NUTSHELL

- *Choose breads or cereals made with one starch: wheat, rye, etc. (Group B).*

- *Many breads and cereals have honey and/or fruits in them and thus would not combine with cooked food (Group A) or milk (Group F). Read the labels.*

- *Eat vegetables raw, sautéed with onions and garlic in olive oil or butter, or steamed to minimize loss of nutrients through cooking.*

- *Never eat dessert! If you are still hungry after a cooked meal, eat more of the cooked meal instead.*

CHAPTER 7:

Beyond the First Three Phases of the Gracie Diet

Now that you are in the habit of spacing meals, avoiding desserts and sodas, and limiting yourself to a single starch, it's time to implement the concept of proper combinations.

Don't Be Afraid to Ask for the Best

Our family prepares our meals at home where we can guarantee the quality, sanitation, and proper preparation of our food. To put it bluntly, I'm uncomfortable having strangers prepare my meals for me, especially since I have worked in a restaurant and am familiar with the many opportunities to cut corners. Nevertheless, you may have no choice but to eat out, so it's important that we address your options.

The first step is to ensure that you are eating high-quality food. The sooner you become selective about the quality of the food you eat, the better for you. Regardless of quality, you will feel better if you properly combine foods. In fact, properly combining lower-quality foods is better for you than improperly combining high-quality foods. But, properly combining high-quality foods is the best of all options. Good food is that which is organically grown free of pesticides, genetic modifications, preservatives, artificial flavorings, and other additives. Bad food is everything else.

Let's consider two types of chicken and cheese sandwiches. You could have a sandwich made with a free-ranging chicken that spent its days pecking and smiling until it naturally reached an ideal weight before finding its way to your lunch plate. Or, you could make a meal of the chicken that was quickly fattened by forced-feeding loads of hormones while it spent its mercifully short life trapped in a cage until it was ready for shipping to your local restaurant or supermarket. You could choose cheese produced from the milk of hormone-free cows that roam the vast pastures, drink unpolluted waters, and are loved by the farmer (who calls them by name and milks them by hand every day). Or, you could choose the cheese from the cows that were fed hormone-laden grain to produce mass volumes of milk to which the dairy added all kinds of chemicals and colorings. You could select bread made from high-quality whole wheat, grown under the golden sun of beautiful plains, or the cheap bleached white bread loaded with chemicals. You could opt for organic lettuce in those fancy plastic cases with the roots intact to preserve freshness and a validation date stamped on the label, or you could choose the other kind...

For that matter, why eat meat at all? A variety of scientific studies claim that humans are not supposed to eat meat or even fish. Some religions call it murder! Who knows for sure? Where do we draw the line? Anyway, you get the idea. Draw your own line and become as strict as you want to be. As your understanding of the basics improves, I encourage you to do your own research and study in order to optimize your healthy eating habits. For now, let's focus on the basic combination principles.

Your Guide to Food Combinations

In the following pages, you'll be introduced to the food groups and food combining principles that are the foundation of the Gracie Diet. The key thing to understand is that the food combination guidelines are not based on taste, appearance, or biological classification, but on what pairings will optimize the digestive process and lead to increased energy, health, and longevity. If the table seems overwhelming at first, don't worry. In the later chapters of this book, I will provide lots of real life examples that will clarify the combination guidelines, as well as an easy-to-follow integration plan so that you can adopt the Gracie Diet with ease.

THE GRACIE DIET TABLE

GROUP A	Foods that combine with each other and one of Group B.

VEGETABLES & GREENS

Artichokes	Cilantro	Okra
Arugula	Corn – Fresh	Onions
Asparagus	Cucumbers	Oregano
Basil	Eggplants	Parsley
Bay Leaves	Endive	Peas - Fresh
Beets - Red	Garlic	Pumpkin
Bell Peppers	Ginger	Radish
Broccoli	Green Beans	Spinach
Brussels Sprouts	Green Onions	Soy - Fresh
Butternut Squash	Hearts of Palm	Turnip
Cabbage	Kale	Tomatoes - Sweet
Carrots	Leeks	Watercress
Cauliflower	Lettuce	Zucchini
Celery	Mushrooms	

MEATS & SEAFOOD

Chicken	Fish Eggs	Red Meat
Crab	Lobster	Shellfish
Crawfish	Mussels	Shrimp
Eggs	Octopus	Squid
Fish	Oysters	

FATS & OILY FOODS

Avocados	Cocoa	Olive Oil
Almonds	Fats in General	Peanuts
Butter / Margarine	Hazelnuts	Pine Nuts
Brazilian Nuts	Melted Cheeses	Sesame Seeds
Cashews	Nuts in General	Walnuts
Coconut - Dried	Olives	Wheat Germ

THE GRACIE DIET TABLE

GROUP B	*Starches* do not combine with each other.

Barley	Dry Peas	Quinoa
Breadfruit	Dry Soy	Rice
Cereals in General	Lentils	Rye
Chestnuts	Manioc	Sweet Potatoes
Dry Beans	Oats	Wheat and Derivatives
Dry Corn/Flour	Potatoes	Yams

GROUP C	*Foods that combine with each other and with one of Group B, if not prepared with fat.*

Apples* - Red	Guava*	Watermelon
Açaí	Honey	All Fresh
Bananas - Dried,	Jaca Fruit	Sweet Fruits
Baked or Cooked	Melons	
Cherimoya*	Papaya	Teas of Leaves or
Cheese - Fresh	Pears - Sweet	Peel of: Orange, Lemon, Apple,
Coconuts - Fresh	Persimmons	Fig Leaves, Black
Cottage Cheese	Plums* - Sweet	Tea, Mate, Cider,
Cream Cheese	Prunes	Chamomile, Various Herbs, etc.
Monterey Jack	Raisins	
Dates	Ricotta Cheese	
Figs - Fresh	Sugar Cane	
Grapes* - Sweet	Sugar in General	

These are sub-acidic fruits and should not be eaten with each other

THE GRACIE DIET TABLE

GROUP D	*Acidic Fruits* do not combine with each other or with anything else.

Apples - Green	Kiwis	Plums - Acidic
Apricots	Lemons	Pomegranate
Blackberries	Lime	Quince
Blueberries	Mangos	Raspberries
Cherries	Oranges	Strawberries
Currants	Peaches	Tangerines
Grapes - Acidic	Pears - Acidic	Tomatoes - Acidic
Grapefruit	Pineapples	All Acidic Fruits

GROUP E	*Raw Bananas*

Combine With:		Do Not Combine With:	
Apples - Red	Papaya	Avocados	Sugar Cane
Cheese - Fresh	Pears - Sweet	Dried Fruits	Oil / Fat in
Cream - Fresh	Watermelon	Honey	General
Grapes - Sweet	All Fresh Sweet	Oily Fruits	All of Group A
Melons	Fruits	Sugar in General	or B
Milk			

GROUP F	*Milk*

Combine With:		Do Not Combine With:	
Bananas - Raw or Baked	Milk Derivatives Except: Curdled Milk, Kefir, Yogurt, and Other Curdled Dairy Products, Which Should Be Eaten Alone.	Avocados	Oily Fruits
Cooked Yolk		Egg Whites	Olives
Artificial Sweeteners		Fruits in General	Sugar in General
All of Group B		Meats in General	All of Group A
		Oils and Fats	

OBSERVATIONS:

Author's Note:

The original table of combinations which Uncle Carlos developed, included "Group G" which explained the proper combinations for "fresh milk cream," the kind we found on dairy farms in the old days. However, unless you have a cow in your backyard, it is virtually impossible to find the kind of fresh milk cream that he was referring to, since everything is processed before it is available to the public. Therefore, I decided to leave Group G out. Also, for the purpose of the Diet, you should treat the "milk cream" that you will find in stores as milk.

Gracie Diet Combination Summary

The Gracie Diet is very simple, but I realize that until you get some real life practice, the table of foods can be quite intimidating. Here's all you really need to know. Aside from an occasional meal that includes acidic fruits (Group D), raw bananas (Group E) or milk (Group F), each of which has their own very specific combination rules (see table above), almost all meals are either Group A based or Group C based. To keep things simple, at home we refer to our Group A meals as "cooked" meals, even though many of the foods in Group A are not actually cooked, and we refer to Group C meals as our "sweet" meals, even though not all foods in Group C are sweet. Just remember, in a Group A meal you can have any combination of the Group A foods together – vegetables, meats, fats, etc. – and one starch from Group B. In a Group C meal you can have any combination of the Group C foods together – sweet fruits, cheeses, etc. – as well as one starch from Group B, as long as the starch is not prepared in fat (oil, butter, etc). Most importantly, in no case shall you ever combine Group A with Group C.

Neutral Foods

Raw or cooked egg yolk, coconut water, brewer's yeast, coffee, and several kinds of tea are considered neutral and compatible with any food.

Coffee

Because the Gracie Diet enables your body to use less energy for digestion, you may find that the extra boost you once sought from caffeine is no longer necessary to start your day. If you enjoy the taste of coffee, you may still drink it. Remember to avoid sweetening your coffee with natural sugar as it does not combine with foods prepared with fat such as oil or butter. If necessary, use an artificial sweetener, but know that some of them may be harmful to your health.

Breads

Bread should be made from whole flour and should not be consumed within 24 hours of being baked. Then, prior to being eaten, it should be toasted or oven-warmed.

Avoid

Sweets, canned foods in syrup, pepper, clover, cinnamon, pickles and vinegar.

Never Eat

Don't eat pork in any form.

Fasting

Before we leave the topic of eating all these foods, we need to talk about NOT eating any food at all – fasting. Carlos Gracie believed that fasting for 24 hours once every month was a good practice, especially for people over the age of forty, as the process allowed the body to cleanse itself. He would have dinner, go to sleep, and then not eat or drink anything until the following evening. After 24 hours, he would take half a watermelon, scoop pieces with a spoon, chew and suck the juice, and spit out the pulp. I believe that Uncle Carlos was right.

For more than ten years, I have fasted once a month. I fast on a day when I know the physical workload will be light, usually on a weekend or in conjunction with travel. I prefer to begin fasting after the second meal of the day because it's usually my heaviest meal and includes cooked foods. Then, all I have to do is skip dinner, go to sleep, and the next morning skip breakfast. It's important to break your fast with fruits, the purest kind of food. After 24 hours without eating or drinking, you've lost body fluids, so a juicy fruit like watermelon is a great way to replenish yourself. The only time I feel hungry is about five hours after the last meal. I push through the hunger pangs by reminding myself that it's only for one day and a delicious fruit meal awaits me.

Dieting is hard; fasting is even harder. But, the results are worth the effort. The first time you fast the enemy within will use every technique in his arsenal to dissuade you. Remember, he has grown accustomed to mixes of foods that may taste good and satisfy your cravings, but ultimately undermine your health and well-being. So, it's normal to feel a strong reaction to your attempts to change your eating habits and flush your digestive system. You're especially vulnerable to making poor food choices when you're hungry, so be ready for the enemy's best moves – hunger pangs and cravings. If you feel that you just can't beat it, then compromise by drinking water. Over time, you will grow accustomed to the initial discomfort of fasting and learn that it quickly passes, especially if you can focus on something other than eating.

I urge you to try fasting. Gandhi fasted for weeks at a time, millions do it every day all over the world – some by choice and others out of necessity, and I do it every month. Just do it. You will feel a couple of inches taller, a couple of pounds lighter, and worth an extra million bucks! You should not fast if you are pregnant, breastfeeding, or taking medicine. A long-term University of Wisconsin study lead by Professor Richard Weindruch, released in July 2009, revealed that rhesus monkeys (chosen for their similarity to humans) with reduced calorie diets were significantly healthier with fewer cases of diabetes, heart and brain disease, and cancer, and thereby lived a longer, more vital life. Fasting is a great habit to develop. It does wonders for your health – and for your mind. When you detach from eating simply as a habit you discover a surprising truth: Sometimes the best meal is the one you don't eat!

Eating Every Other Day

Mark Mattson, a researcher at the National Institute on Aging in Baltimore, Maryland, thinks an alternate route may be through what he calls intermittent fasting. Health benefits in mice that eat only every other day are similar to those for mice that eat a calorie-restricted diet—they live 30 percent longer, Mattson says. And, he adds, "We see vast improvements in variables that indicate risk of disease." Mattson's objective is not weight loss (though the ad hoc fasters happily report pounds lost, as well as other health benefits including reduced allergy sensitivity and more energy). Nor is Mattson especially interested in extending life span. Instead, he wants to boost what he calls the human "health span"—the period of a life in which a person enjoys good health, even into their eighties or nineties.

Points to Remember:

- Whenever possible, opt for organic and minimally processed foods. It's an investment that will pay off in a longer, healthier life.

- Initially, you may need to reference the Gracie Diet Table whenever you are unsure of what group a food belongs to. Eventually, it will become second nature to you.

- After age 40, consider fasting for one day each month, and always break your fast with a fruit meal.

 THE GRACIE DIET IN A NUTSHELL

- *Foods prepared with fat/oil/butter do not combine with the sugar in desserts such as cookies, ice cream, or even fruit.*

- *If you have a sweet tooth, satisfy your cravings by making a meal from Group C.*

- *To lose weight, eat a one-fruit meal. Start with one meal per week, and gradually increase to once a day. Remember to alternate the fruits.*

- *Do not eat the same food within a 24-hour period.*

CHAPTER 8:

The Gracie Diet on the Go

How to Eat Healthily When You're on the Run

Knowing what to order when eating out can make a huge difference in your health. In this section, we'll see how to order from some popular restaurants and fast food chains. Note that I included this chapter to demonstrate how the Gracie Diet can accommodate familiar eating patterns and habits, not to endorse eating in restaurants. I have eaten in a few of these places and I know I am better off if I never repeat that mistake. However, if you have no choice, there are ways to order food that can make the meal less harmful. I will show you how to order and how to avoid the common mistakes that will make a big difference.

It can be difficult to order plain food. Ordering a salad with some pasta and a piece of fish seems simple enough. However, when they add the dressing to the salad, the sauce over the pasta, and a squeeze of lemon over your fish, it changes everything! That is enough to transform what could have been a harmless meal into something that is actually harmful to your health. You have options.

When away from home, go to the local supermarket and get some seasonal fruits, like a few ripe bananas and some red delicious apples or a slice of watermelon. If you know you're going to be out and about at mealtime, take your fruits with you. Plan ahead and you can't go wrong! If you don't have access to a market, then try to order food that you can "simplify." I rarely eat at fast food restaurants, but a few years ago during a long trip I stopped at a restaurant of a popular chain to use the restroom. Because it was way past my time to eat and I had no other options, I ordered a couple of fish filet sandwiches with no sauce, no pickles, and a glass of water. No matter where you are, there is always a way to improvise.

Another challenge you'll face in a restaurant is food quality. I'm not talking about taste or portion, but the freshness and purity of the food. Clearly, a restaurant exists to make a profit. Their balance sheet determines the quality of food they will use, and with rare exceptions, the quality will vary from bad to worse. From the kind of lettuce to the quality of the meat and the type of bread, everything is calculated to make it affordable to all and by doing so generate a bigger profit for them. Every month, approximately 9 out of 10 American children visit a McDonald's restaurant. In 1970, Americans spent about $6 billion on fast food. In 2006, the spending rose to nearly $142 billion.

The problem is that your health is not a priority in the cost-profit equation. Since nothing impacts your health like the food you eat, you can't ignore the fact that it is your responsibility to make the right choices. You must look out for your health and that of your loved ones, because nobody else will.

Learn the Gracie Diet Food Selection Process

When ordering at a familiar restaurant, you probably know what you want. Based on your choice of entrée, you can build the rest of your meal. Follow this process:

Suppose you're considering a dish of fish, rice, and vegetables. That means you can't eat the wheat bread the waiter will bring to the table because it does not combine with rice (both are in Group B: Starches and therefore do not combine with one another). You could, however, eat the bread if you substitute rice for the pasta with the fish and vegetables, because the pasta and the bread are both made out of wheat (Group B). Just be sure to verify that there are no potatoes mixed in with the vegetables since they are a different starch (Group B) and do not combine with wheat either. If you order a salad, use no dressing other than olive oil and salt.

Many appetizers are acceptable – Carpaccio, crab cakes, spinach artichoke dip, avocado egg rolls, etc. Once again, you must think about the meal as a whole, and be sure to ask what the spinach artichoke dip is served with. If it's served with bread, it means that it's OK with the pasta from the entrée since they are both made from the same starch – wheat (Group B). If it's served with corn or potato chips instead, since they are different starches, it would not combine. The same principle applies to egg rolls. The wrap is made with wheat, so you're OK if you've ordered pasta.

Learn to drink only water without lemon or lime. If you enjoy carbonation, then drink sparkling water instead of soda.

Finally, never eat dessert!

How Well Do You Know the Combinations?

This section will help determine your understanding of the Gracie Diet Table of food combining. Feel free to check the table as you analyze the options. In the following 10 sets find the one food that does not combine with all the others:

1.
a) Mashed potatoes
b) French fries
c) Rice
d) Baked potatoes
e) Turkey

2.
a) Eggs
b) Bread
c) Beef
d) Pasta
e) They all combine.

3.
a) Potato chips
b) Tuna sandwich
c) Pizza
d) Cheeseburger
e) Spaghetti

4.
a) Cantaloupe
b) Watermelon
c) Sweet pears
d) Blueberries
e) Bananas

5.
a) Honeydew melon
b) Persimmons
c) Green apples
d) Papaya
e) Honey

6.
a) Wheat bread
b) Watermelon juice
c) Guava jelly
d) Peanut butter
e) Monterey Jack cheese

7.
a) Bananas
b) Red apples
c) Cantaloupe
d) Kiwi
e) Papaya

8.
a) Pickles
b) Broccoli
c) Spinach
d) Cucumber
e) Potatoes

9.
a) Fish
b) Bacon
c) Chicken
d) Beef
e) Rice

10.
a) Sparkling water
b) Carrot juice
c) Coconut water
d) Coffee
e) They all combine.

In the next 10 sets, identify which meal violates the Gracie Diet combination guidelines.

11.

a) Rice, salmon, broccoli, cashews, carrot juice
b) Spaghetti, chicken, green beans, pizza, coconut water
c) Baked potatoes, French fries, lettuce, eggs
d) Beans, rice, turkey, squash, sparking water
e) They all combine.

12.

a) Watermelon juice, crackers, and Jack cheese
b) Cantaloupe juice, raisin bread, and cream cheese
c) Orange juice, wheat toast, and cottage cheese
d) Bananas, cream cheese, and red apples
e) They all combine.

13.

a) Cheeseburger, scrambled eggs, salad, and water
b) Pizza, avocado, chicken, sparkling water
c) Steak, rice, vegetables, coffee
d) Fish, spaghetti, green beans, lemonade
e) They all combine.

14.

a) Corn soup, grilled cheese sandwich, coconut water
b) Grilled chicken, pasta, avocado, fruit salad
c) Salmon, quinoa, broccoli, carrot juice
d) Sautéed vegetables, rice, beef, salad
e) They all combine.

15.

a) Peanut butter, jelly, bread, apple juice
b) Seafood risotto, squash, chamomile tea
c) Pizza, avocado, chicken, angel hair pasta, coffee
d) Black beans, green beans, walnuts, water
e) They all combine.

16.
a) Vegetables, rice, avocado, cashews, ice tea (no sugar)
b) Fish, spaghetti, carrots, broccoli, water
c) Chicken, pasta, salad, pistachios, sparkling water
d) Beef, mashed potatoes, celery, coconut water
e) They all combine.

17.
a) Rice, shrimp, vegetables, coconut water
b) Pizza, avocado, French fries, carrot juice
c) Baked potatoes, grilled halibut, asparagus, water
d) Pasta, chicken, salad, cashews, sparkling water
e) They all combine.

18.
a) Lettuce, cucumber, bell peppers, radish, vinegar
b) Spinach, heart of palm, cashews, olive oil, salt
c) Romaine lettuce, onions, olives, avocado, bell peppers
d) Arugula, broccoli, beets, celery, spinach
e) They all combine.

19.
a) Fish and chips
b) Macaroni and cheese
c) Hamburger and French fries
d) Bagels and coffee
e) They all combine.

20.
a) Cantaloupe, sweet pears, Monterey Jack cheese
b) Papaya, dates, cottage cheese
c) Honeydew melon, fresh figs, cream cheese
d) Watermelon, mangos, cottage cheese
e) Apples, bananas, cream cheese

Correct Answers:

1-c) Potatoes and Rice (Group B) are different starches and do not combine.

2-e) They all combine.

3-a) Wheat and Potatoes (Group B) are different starches and do not combine.

4-d) Blueberries (Group D) are acidic and do not combine with anything else.

5-c) Green apples (Group D) are acidic and do not combine with anything else.

6-d) Peanut butter (Group A) does not combine with fruits or sweets (Group C).

7-d) Kiwi (Group D) is acidic and should not be consumed with anything else.

8-a) Pickles are fermented cucumbers preserved in vinegar. They do not combine.

9-b) Bacon or any form of pork meat should never be consumed.

10-e) They all combine.

11-d) Beans and rice (Group B) are both starches and do not combine.

12-c) Orange juice (Group D) is acidic and does not combine with anything else.

13-d) Lemon (Group D) is acidic and does not combine with anything else.

14-b) Chicken and avocado (Group A) do not combine with fruits (Groups C or D).

15-a) Peanut butter (Group A) does not combine with sweets (Group C).

16-e) They all combine.

17-b) Pizza (wheat) and potatoes (Group B) are starches and do not combine.

18-a) Vinegar and all other spices do not combine and should be avoided.

19-c) The bun (wheat) and potatoes (Group B) are starches and don't combine.

20-d) Mango (Group D) is acidic and it should only be eaten by itself.

Real Life Examples Drawn from the Menus of Popular Restaurants

Following are several samples of Group A meals from popular restaurants. A "*NOTE*" follows each of them suggesting the best way to order the dish to meet the combination requirements for the Gracie Diet.

WARNING: In many restaurants, the waiter will bring a basket of bread and butter to your table. Remember, the bread is made of wheat (Group B). So, you should only eat it if you plan on ordering an entrée that will combine with it.

CHEESECAKE FACTORY

AVOCADO EGGROLLS

Avocado, sun-dried tomato, red onion, and cilantro deep fried in a crisp Chinese wrapper. Served with a dipping sauce.

NOTE: *Because the wrapper is made of wheat, you should plan on eating pasta as part of your entrée. Do not touch the sauce.*

MINI CRABCAKES

Louisiana crab served with mustard and tartar sauce.

NOTE: *Enjoy them without the mustard or tartar sauce.*

CHOPPED SALAD

Romaine lettuce, grilled chicken, tomato, avocado, corn, bacon, blue cheese, apple, and vinaigrette.

NOTE: *Ask for no tomatoes, bacon, blue cheese, apple slices, or vinaigrette.*

REMEMBER: Drink water, sparkling water, or tea without lemon or sugar. And no dessert!

LUAU SALAD

Grilled chicken breast with mixed greens, cucumbers, green onions, red and yellow peppers, green beans, mango, and wontons with macadamia nuts and sesame seeds. Tossed in vinaigrette.

NOTE: The mango and the vinaigrette must be removed from this salad. You need to make sure the wontons, which are made from wheat, will combine with the starch in the main entrée.

FACTORY BURRITO GRANDE

Burrito with chicken, cheese, rice, onions, and peppers, topped with guacamole, sour cream, and salsa. Served with black beans and rice.

NOTE: Classic example of too many starches (Group B) in one meal; wheat tortilla, rice, and beans, which is not good. We can only eat one. (Also, avocado is OK but guacamole usually has lemon juice which is not OK. Sour cream and salsa are to be avoided.) There is a lot to take out!

ORANGE CHICKEN

Deep fried chicken breast in a sweet and spicy orange sauce. Served over white rice and garnished with vegetables.

NOTE: Deep fried is tolerable, so here is the problem – "sweet and spicy orange sauce." Also, keep in mind that if you decide to choose the rice, you should pass on the complimentary wheat bread.

CRUSTED CHICKEN ROMANO

Breast of chicken coated with a Romano and Parmesan cheese crust. Served with pasta in tomato sauce.

NOTE: Although tomatoes are acidic, if cooked, tomato sauce is OK. As an alternative, you may ask for olive oil and garlic on your pasta. You may have the complimentary bread and butter since the bread and pasta are made from the same starch – wheat. You can have a salad (no salad dressing; olive oil and salt instead) and/ or crab cakes as an appetizer, but stay away from the spicy sauce that comes with it.

REMEMBER: Drink water, sparkling water, or tea without lemon or sugar. And no dessert!

CHICKEN MADEIRA

Sautéed chicken breast topped with asparagus and melted mozzarella cheese, with mushroom Madeira sauce. Served with mashed potatoes.

NOTE: *If you want to have bread and butter or avocado egg rolls as an appetizer, you must substitute the mashed potatoes for spaghetti with garlic and olive oil, since potatoes do not combine with bread or the egg rolls' flour wrapper, which are made from wheat. You may have a salad but remember to stay away from the dressing, pepper, etc., and use olive oil and salt only.*

SHRIMP SCAMPI

Sautéed with garlic, white wine, olive oil, basil, parsley, and tomato. Served with angel hair pasta.

NOTE: *Be sure to ask for no lemon or pepper. You may have the bread and butter that they will put on your table, since bread and pasta are made from the same starch – wheat. You may have a salad and/or avocado egg rolls since they are wrapped in wheat flour tortillas.*

MISO SALMON

With vegetables and steamed rice.

NOTE: *No bread or avocado egg rolls, since they are made with wheat and do not combine with rice. If you want to have the warm bread and butter that they will bring to the table or if you're thinking about ordering the avocado egg rolls, you should have pasta instead of rice, or ask for the salmon on a bed of spinach (without rice). Either way, you may have a salad. No dressing though, olive oil and salt only.*

FILET MIGNON

Served with French fries and onion strings.

NOTE: *French fries are made from potatoes, so, do not combine with the complimentary bread, the avocado egg rolls, or the salad's croutons, since they are all made out of wheat. If you want to have those, you should ask for pasta which is also made out of wheat, instead of the fries.*

REMEMBER: *Drink water, sparkling water, or tea without lemon or sugar. And no dessert!*

GRILLED CHICKEN AND AVOCADO CLUB

Grilled chicken breast with avocado, bacon, tomato, melted Swiss cheese, and herb mayonnaise. Served with French fries.

NOTE: In this sandwich, request no bacon, tomato, or mayonnaise. Also, leave out the French fries (potatoes), since they don't combine with the bread (wheat).

CHICKEN, MUSHROOM, AND ROASTED GARLIC PIZZA

With grilled onions, mozzarella, and Parmesan.

NOTE: You may have the bread and butter, since the bread and pizza are made from the same starch – wheat. You may also have a salad. No dressing though, olive oil and salt only.

ROASTED VEGETABLES AND GOAT CHEESE PIZZA

With roasted Japanese eggplant, red and yellow peppers, grilled onion, artichokes, olives, tomato, and mozzarella.

NOTE: You may have the bread and butter, since the bread and the pasta are made from the same starch – wheat. You may have a salad and/or crab cakes (no sauce) and/or avocado egg rolls since they are wrapped in wheat flour tortillas.

CALIFORNIA PIZZA KITCHEN

PIZZA MARGHERITA

Italian tomatoes and fresh mozzarella cheeses with fresh basil and Parmesan cheese.

NOTE: Tomatoes are acidic, but if they are cooked, it's OK to leave them in. I often ask to add an avocado. A green salad is always a good idea and you know the deal, no dressing; olive oil and salt only.

ROASTED GARLIC CHICKEN PIZZA

Garlic, grilled chicken, mozzarella cheese, onions, and parsley with white wine and garlic-shallot butter.

NOTE: Although chicken is included in Group A and would combine, I usually substitute it with avocado. Sometimes I have an artichoke dip with pita bread or maybe even a side order of broccoli.

REMEMBER: Drink water, sparkling water, or tea without lemon or sugar. And no dessert!

GRILLED VEGETARIAN SANDWICH

Mushrooms, grilled red and yellow peppers with melted fontina and mozzarella cheeses, baby field greens, sliced Roma tomatoes, and sun-dried tomato aioli. Served with bread: herb-onion focaccia or garlic-cheese focaccia.

NOTE: If you want to ask for a salad, get it without dressing. Use olive oil and salt only.

APPLEBEE'S

MOZZARELLA STICKS

Fried and served with marinara sauce.

NOTE: Tomatoes are acidic, but because they are cooked, it's OK to eat them.

DYNAMITE SHRIMP

Shrimp coated in bread crumbs and fried, then tossed in a spicy sauce.

NOTE: Request "sauce on the side" so that you don't have to eat it. Also, since it's prepared with bread crumbs (wheat), you need to make sure it combines with the starch in the main entrée.

GRILLED CHICKEN CAESAR SALAD

Chicken breast atop a bed of romaine lettuce tossed in garlic Caesar dressing. Topped with challah croutons and shaved Parmesan cheese.

NOTE: Ask for the Caesar dressing on the side and use a minimum amount until you can wean yourself away from it and start using only olive oil and salt. Again, remember that if you want to eat croutons (wheat) you need to make sure it combines with the starch in the main entrée.

BOURBON STREET STEAK

Steak with Cajun spices and served with sautéed onions and mushrooms.

NOTE: Ask for no Cajun spices. It will pay off in the long run. It's much healthier to eat natural foods with no spices at all.

REMEMBER: Drink water, sparkling water, or tea without lemon or sugar. And no dessert!

STEAK AND PORTOBELLO

Grilled sirloin steak with sliced, sautéed Portobello mushrooms and brown sauce paired with steamed herb potatoes and seasonal vegetables.

NOTE: Remember to pass on the savory brown sauce! Also, potatoes do not combine with the salad's croutons, or the wheat bread that may be brought to your table, or any other Group B foods.

FRIED CHICKEN

Chicken breast, lightly breaded in seasonings. Served with garlic mashed potatoes, gravy, and seasonal vegetables.

NOTE: The breaded (wheat) chicken does not combine with mashed potatoes. You shouldn't eat the gravy, either. You should cancel the potatoes and ask for pasta which is made out of wheat.

FISH AND CHIPS

Whitefish fillets, dipped in a light batter and fried; served with fries, cole slaw, and tartar sauce.

NOTE: Forget about cole slaw and tartar sauce; pretend they are not even there. We've got to learn to enjoy the "natural" taste of all foods.

CHICKEN BROCCOLI PASTA ALFREDO BOWL

Grilled or blackened chicken on fettuccine tossed with broccoli and creamy Alfredo sauce. Topped with Parmesan and served with toasted bread.

NOTE: Ask for olive oil (and garlic if you like it!) instead of the Alfredo sauce which is prepared with milk and cream, thus not a good combination. Cream does not combine with meat.

GRILLED SHRIMP PESTO ALFREDO FETTUCCINE

Shrimp tossed with spices and served with basil pesto Alfredo fettuccine, grape tomatoes, and Italian cheeses; with shaved Parmesan and toasted bread.

NOTE: Tell them to 'keep it real' and avoid any spices or tomatoes. It's best to avoid all spices.

REMEMBER: Drink water, sparkling water, or tea without lemon or sugar. And no dessert!

BREWTUS STEAK BURGER™

Ten ounces of chopped sirloin burger, topped with cheddar cheese and smoked bacon, and served on a toasted bun.

NOTE: Insist on "no smoked bacon." Never eat pork!

Most of the burgers and sandwiches include fries.

NOTE: Just because they include French fries doesn't mean you must eat them with your sandwich. Having the fries (potato) with bread (wheat) is a Group B combination conflict that should be avoided.

SUBWAY

Tuna or turkey, cheese, lettuce, olives, avocado, and onions on bread.

NOTE: Never add sauces, mayonnaise, pepper, vinegar, ketchup, pickles, and of course, never eat pork.

MCDONALD'S

Cheeseburger, Fillet-O-Fish, or chicken breast sandwich.

NOTE: Don't eat fries if you want to eat bread. The idea is to choose between wheat or potatoes. If you do want to have French fries (potatoes), you may have the hamburger patty, the fish fillet, or the chicken breast and the other ingredients (lettuce, onions, and melted cheese) but no wheat bun. Be sure to request no pickles or sauce/dressing. It's better to have two hamburgers than one hamburger with French fries.

Side Salad

Salad Mix: Iceberg lettuce, romaine lettuce, spring mix (may contain baby red romaine, baby green romaine, baby red leaf, baby green leaf, baby red Swiss chard, baby red oak, baby green oak, lolla rossa, tango, tatsoi, arugula, mizuna, radicchio, frisee), carrots, and grape tomatoes.

NOTE: Be sure to insist on no dressing or seasonings. Also, take out the tomatoes, as they are acidic. Chicken is optional but bacon isn't, so stay away from it. Remember, never eat pork!

REMEMBER: Drink water, sparkling water, or tea without lemon or sugar. And no dessert!

Improvise Anywhere

The Diet is flexible enough that, even if you are at a 7-Eleven in the middle of nowhere, you can still improvise. Here are some suggestions: First - look for any fresh fruit and use it as the base of your meal, taking into consideration the proper combinations; Second - if there are no fresh fruits, try a salad (no dressing) and nuts (without raisins); Third - a bag of nuts (without raisins) and water, crackers are optional and finally – a tuna or turkey sandwich and water.

Points to Remember:

• You can still follow the Gracie Diet when you're eating out.

• Although the food quality may be inferior, you can minimize the harm of restaurant food by modifying your selection to comply with the Gracie Diet.

• Only eat the bread in the basket if you know that the starch in your main course will also be wheat derived.

 THE GRACIE DIET IN A NUTSHELL

• *Use only olive oil as a salad dressing. Salt may be added for taste.*
• *Always eat salad first.*
• *If you miss the carbonation from sodas, drink sparkling water instead.*
• *Remember that children will drink what you put in the refrigerator.*

CHAPTER 9:

Tips for Losing Weight

To optimize digestion, increase energy, and have a long healthy life, you must space your meals appropriately and properly combine your foods at each sitting. However, if weight loss is your primary goal, you will need to go one step further. You will need to control your caloric intake and minimize the consumption of certain foods, and in order to do that you will need to develop a very high level of self-control.

How Dieting Helps You to Acquire the Gracie "Iron Will"

The Gracie Diet is a great opportunity to develop the priceless habit of self-discipline. I learned from my father at an early age that every meal was a chance to practice self-control. Sometimes it was a question of me having three slices of toast instead of four. Or two scoops of ice cream instead of three. Why not one more slice of toast or another scoop of ice cream? Because you're no longer hungry! When I felt like overeating, more often than not I was being led by the anticipation of how good the food would taste. In other words *pleasure* was the driving force behind that extra slice or the extra scoop. There came a time when I could tell myself: "Okay, I will have another slice and one more scoop – but not today!" That was a major revelation. Confronting the temptation and then denying it caused the craving to vanish. It made me stronger. It put me in control. It increased my self-worth. Not only is this self-mastery the single most important element of the weight-loss equation, but it will positively impact every aspect of your life.

Calorie Control

Calories are measurements of energy: 3,500 calories equals one pound of fat. So, burning 3,500 calories means losing one pound of fat. When it comes to weight loss, there is one more equation that matters: You must burn more calories than you consume. Men between the ages of 19-50 should consume between 2,200 and 2,600 calories per day. Women 19-50 should consume between 1,800 and 2,200 per day. The more active you are, the higher your metabolism will be, and the more calories you will burn.

John O. Holloszy of the Washington University School of Medicine, in St. Louis, Missouri, and his colleagues cataloged what they call "profound and sustained beneficial effects" of the calorie-restricted diet. The dietitian-approved meal plan was enlivened by a nutrient-dense array of fruits, vegetables, legumes, and whole grains (*Proceedings of the National Academies of Sciences*).

"The calorie-restriction subjects scored vastly better on all major risk factors for heart disease including total cholesterol, triglycerides, and blood pressure. Each of these tends to increase with advancing age. They also have very low amounts of body fat compared to the average person in the control group, who had about 25 percent body fat. This quality protects the calorie restrictors from the type 2 diabetes associated with obesity," Holloszy says.

Play This Game at Your Next Meal

As a great way to begin developing your discipline while monitoring your food consumption, do this at your next meal. Find something that you really enjoy eating and tell yourself, "I will only eat half of it!" If you can "win" this game, you will take a major step forward in developing your personal discipline and healthy eating habits. You'll be amazed at how easily you can trim your meals and achieve great results with less food. A good rule to adhere to is to stop eating when you are 80% full. Just remember, you'll be eating again in about 4 ½ hours anyway. Eating less at each meal is good for your body and your mind! I can't overemphasize enough how practicing dietary discipline will enhance your overall health. You simply won't believe how it will improve your ability to achieve your personal goals.

A Surefire Way to Burn Fat

In addition to monitoring your caloric intake, one great way to help you reach your weight-loss goal is to make one-fruit-meals part of your routine. Once a day, have a meal in which you limit yourself to a single fruit. You may have as much of the one fruit as you want, but you must eat only the one fruit – without bread or cheese. Be sure to eat enough to tide you over until the next meal. This may take some practice, since most people aren't accustomed to eating four or five bananas or half a watermelon in one sitting. Since you are only eating one kind of fruit, you may feel hungry before the 4 ½ hours are up. No worries - drink a glass of water and your hunger pangs will subside! Your body will soon grow accustomed to the regimen. Remember: Don't have the same fruit again for 24 hours.

Managing Your Carbohydrates

The extreme popularity of the Atkins, South Beach, and other low-carbohydrate diets led many people to believe that carbohydrates are the primary cause of the obesity epidemic. That's a dangerous oversimplification, similar to "fat is bad." Don't be misled by these broad pronouncements on the dangers of carbohydrates. They are an extremely important part of a healthy diet. Carbohydrates are the most common source of energy found in food, and they are vital in promoting proper organ function. The key is to understand the difference between complex carbohydrates or "good carbs," and simple carbohydrates, "bad carbs." Easily digestible simple carbohydrates from white bread, white rice, pastries, sugared sodas, and other highly processed foods may, indeed, contribute to weight gain. On the other hand, complex carbohydrates from whole grains, beans, fruits, an vegetables deliver minerals, fiber, and a host of essential vitamins. Stick to minimally processed whole grains, fruits, and vegetables and you'll be good to go!

Protein Sources

Also known as the building block of life, protein's most important role is to build, maintain, and replace tissue in our bodies. Protein is a long chain of amino acids linked together. Our muscles, organs, and some of our hormones are made up of mostly protein. Our body is able to produce some of the amino acids (protein) we need. The rest (known as essential amino acids) must be obtained through our diets. Since I choose not to eat red meat, people often ask where I get my protein. Some of the best sources of protein are: fish, avocados, beans, soy, dairy, nuts, and white meat poultry. In fact, scientific studies have proven repeatedly that a diet derived exclusively from the vegetable kingdom can provide all the essential amino acids for optimal health, which means you can get all the protein you need without the cholesterol that is contained in all animal products.

Critical Fat Facts

Fat is a necessary nutrient and most foods contain some type of fat. Fat helps in our energy production and our blood clotting; it helps regulate blood pressure and to maintain a healthy nervous system; and your skin, hair, and nails all depend on it. But, some fats are better for you than others, so it is critical that you know the difference between healthy, good fats, and unhealthy, bad fats. The good fats include the following: monounsaturated fat (olives, avocados, nuts), polyunsaturated fat (vegetable oils, cereals, bananas, hemp seeds) and omega-3 fatty acids (fish, flax, walnuts). Then there are the bad fats, and they include: saturated fat (animal products such as meat, dairy, and eggs), trans fat (hydrogenated oils found in cookies, crackers, cakes, and also common in fried foods) and cholesterol (animal products, dairy, organs). Although all fats are okay in moderation, if you're trying to lose weight and reach optimum health, it is best to stick to the good fats and minimize the rest.

How to Lose Weight and Still Occasionally Enjoy Alcohol

Alcohol does not exist in the Gracie Diet, but if drinking is part of your lifestyle, you should at least follow the rest of the guidelines. Your eventual goal should be to wean off alcohol altogether, but until that happens, focus on reducing the frequency of your consumption. If you normally drink every weekend, start by cutting it back to every other weekend, and then down to once a month. Eventually, when you begin to feel the positive results of all the other dietary changes you are making, and your confidence is growing from living a healthier lifestyle, you will find greater satisfaction in resisting the temptation than you do from drinking, and that's when you'll be able to quit completely and feel great about it! I can tell you from experience that if you have children, choosing the alcohol-free path will be one of the most important decisions you'll ever make.

How to Stay True to the Gracie Diet

What do you do when someone prepares a meal for you that does not comply with the Gracie Diet? How do you handle a big Thanksgiving dinner full of incompatible food combinations or a celebration where everyone is drinking alcohol (and lots of it)? First, make a positive choice. Follow the course of action that will make you feel good about yourself. If you make an exception to the Gracie dietary guidelines, then do it because you feel that it's the right thing to do. Ask yourself which will make you feel better, avoiding unhealthy food selections or pleasing your host? Of course, you should do it tactfully, respectfully, and confidently. Often, it's easiest for everyone if you just employ a simple excuse – like you're not feeling well or you're allergic to certain foods or beverages. Just be aware that what's at stake here is something much larger than the momentary circumstance. As a child, I never saw my father or other members of my family smoke or drink – and I'm sure they were conscious of the positive influence this would have on me.

Points to Remember:

- It doesn't matter how good your weight-loss plan is, if you don't develop the discipline to make it happen, it's useless.

- If weight loss is your goal, manage your caloric intake and, as a general rule, always leave the table with your body feeling 80% full.

- Besides the health and safety concerns associated with drinking alcohol, remember that if drinking is a part of your lifestyle, eating right is that much more important.

 THE GRACIE DIET IN A NUTSHELL

- *Always chew your food thoroughly. The assimilation of everything your body needs requires that the food literally pass through the walls of the intestine.*

- *During a meal, focus on eating. Avoid reading, talking on the phone, or watching television while you eat.*

- *Eat enough at each meal to hold you over until the next one, but don't stuff yourself.*

- *Stop eating when you're still able to eat more.*

CHAPTER 10:
The Role of Exercise

Physical exercise – and especially its relationship to diet – is an important but commonly misunderstood component of a healthy lifestyle. The most common misconception is that you must adopt a rigorous workout routine in order to lose weight. How the body reacts to different types of exercises depends on many factors. The key is to find the right exercise for you. More is not necessarily better. The idea that weight control is linked to exercise is seemingly obvious. In all areas of our lives, we see that work brings results and hard work usually brings even better results. But with regard to weight control, research proves that more is not better.

Dr. Wayne Miller and colleagues at George Washington University Medical Center conducted a survey of 493 weight-loss studies. The purpose was to determine whether the addition of aerobic exercise to a restricted calorie diet accelerated weight loss. The research showed that diet and moderate aerobic exercise provide only a small improvement in weight loss compared to diet alone. [Source: *http://www.timinvermont.com/fitness/aerobic.htm*]

An Appalachian State University study focused on a group of 91 obese women organized into four groups. The first group followed a restricted diet of 1,200 to 1,300 calories per day; group two had no diet restrictions but performed aerobic exercise for 45 minutes, five days each week; the third group combined exercise and diet. The women in the fourth group acted as controls and followed their normal daily routines. Although they exercised for almost four hours each week, the exercise-only group lost just three pounds. The women combining diet and exercise got the best results, losing a combined 16 pounds of fat. But this was only one pound more than the group on the diet alone. The researchers stated that aerobic exercise had only "minor, insignificant effect" on fat loss. [Source: *International Journal of Sport Nutrition, 8, 213-222*]

For exercise to have a real impact on your weight, you would need to follow a strict regimen for a long time. It's always easier said than done. For most of us, strong intentions and high motivation quickly erode in the face of demanding daily workouts. The good news is that it's not a disaster if you ease up on the exercise, as long as you keep doing something. While diet is more effective than exercise in weight management, it's still important to exercise. The real problems arise only when people completely stop exercising. I offer three points to guide you in whatever exercise program you choose to follow.

Make It Fun

Find an exercise that interests you. The problem with most aerobic workouts is that they are incredibly boring. Few people can sustain the motivation to ride a stationary bicycle or climb a Stairmaster for weeks or months in order to see any benefits. To be sure, some motivate themselves by challenging their bodies and minds to the max in every workout. For elite athletes like Lance Armstrong, exercise means reaching his physical limit and staying there for as long as possible. If he could, he would probably remain at that point all the time. Monotony is not a problem because he turns every session into the Tour de France. But most of us are not elite athletes with the accompanying obsessive mindset. As a result, it's only a matter of time before we burn out. That's why it's best if exercise is a byproduct of an exciting or enjoyable activity instead of the main focus. For example, our training at the Gracie Jiu-Jitsu Academy doesn't include calisthenics or weight-lifting, but the students are shedding pounds without even realizing it because they are so consumed with learning the techniques. Whether you choose jiu-jitsu, basketball, or just a brisk walk through a pleasant neighborhood, the important thing is that it stimulates you beyond the fitness aspect so that you can sustain the activity for a lifetime.

Start Simple

Your exercise should be moderately challenging. The key to weight loss is to find the right balance of time and exertion that you can sustain given your personal schedule, interests, and physical abilities. Workout for as long and as hard as you like, but understand that after approximately the first fifteen minutes, there's a sharp drop off in the positive effects of exercise. Exercising for an hour doesn't mean you'll get twice the effect of exercising for thirty minutes. You will surely benefit, but the return on your effort diminishes over time. It's much more important, therefore, to be consistent and comfortable than to "knock yourself out." I recommend brisk walking, especially with a partner, for weight control and overall health. If you take a thirty-minute walk every day at a fast but comfortable pace, that will give you virtually all the benefits that you'd get from a more strenuous (and less pleasant) workout. And if you take the walk with someone whose company you enjoy, the time will pass very quickly.

Keep Climbing

The real goal of exercising today should be to want to do it again tomorrow. No matter how good a workout is one day – or one week, or even for a whole month – you will lose the benefits unless you continue your exercise over a much longer time period. In fact, your goal should be finding an activity that you can enjoy for the rest of your life. The reason so many people are so passionate about Gracie Jiu-Jitsu is because anyone can do it and you never stop getting better. Even at 95 my father was still experimenting with new techniques! If you already have a regular exercise routine, that's great. If you don't, start with a 20-minute walk three times a week. Keep a calendar of your exercise schedule and increase one digit on either side of your routine every two weeks. From a 20-minute walk three times a week, go to 30 minutes three times a week, or 20 minutes four times a week. Then break up the routine by expanding to include one new exercise – like sit-ups or push-ups – every two weeks. Gradually increase the number of repetitions, and every two weeks add an entirely new exercise. The quick, positive health benefits of this exercise will have you so motivated that you'll be amazed at how much more you want to do. It's definitely a great feeling – but don't just depend on a short-term high. You're not training for a sprint. You're not even training for a marathon. You're training for life – a long, healthy life.

How do supplements work with the Diet?

The purpose of the Gracie Diet is to optimize your health so you don't need supplements. A well-balanced diet with a good variety of fruits and vegetables, nuts and grains will provide all the nutrients you need. Only if you are not getting your daily servings of fruits and vegetables would I recommend looking into a multivitamin supplement. In no case would I recommend the use of a weight-loss or weight-gaining supplement. Although they may help you reach your short-term objective, studies of many such supplements have revealed negative long-term impact on your overall health.

Points to Remember:

- In order to be sustainable, exercise can't be "a means to an end." It should be fun and rewarding in its own right.

- Find an exercise program that's reasonably challenging, not overwhelming.

- If you don't already have a workout routine that you are 100% passionate about, give Gracie Jiu-Jitsu a shot. I guarantee you will not be disappointed. Go to *www.GracieUniversity.com* to watch Gracie Combatives – Lesson 1 for free, and if you like what you see you can find a Certified Training Center near you!

 THE GRACIE DIET IN A NUTSHELL

- *Fast once a month (if over 40 years old).*
- *Choose good quality foods.*
- *Do not smoke.*
- *Do not consume alcohol, sodas, or processed liquids.*
- *Take a 15-30 minute nap every day.*

CHAPTER 11:

The Final Round

Tips and Reminders

- Raw or cooked egg yolk, coconut water, brewer's yeast, coffee, and several kinds of tea are neutral. They're compatible with any food.
- Bread should be made from whole flour and should not be consumed within 24 hours of being baked. Then, prior to being eaten, it should be toasted or oven-warmed.
- Avoid sweets, canned foods in syrup, and spices including: pepper, clove, cinnamon, mustard, pickles, and vinegar.
- Don't eat pork in any form.
- Space meals at least 4½ hours apart to ensure complete digestion before you eat again. It's OK to wait longer. Young children may eat every 4 hours. If you feel hungry before it's time to eat, drink a glass of water. Never snack!

How to Eat Cooked Foods, Vegetables, and Meats (Group A)

- It's best to eat cooked food at home where you can monitor food quality, ensure proper preparation, and guarantee proper hygiene.
- The problem with restaurant food is the heavy use of condiments, spices, and sauces, which change the real taste of the foods and could adversely affect food combinations and meal digestibility.
- When eating out, order the food as plain as possible, always requesting the dressing or sauces on the side so that you can use it less and less, or none at all. It's always better to only use olive oil and salt.

- Eat as many fresh vegetables and dark leafy greens as possible.
- Avoid drinking too much liquid with your meal.
- Try to eat your cooked meal in the afternoon when your metabolism is more active, thereby making it easier to digest.
- In no event shall Group C foods be consumed with Group A.
- When cheese is melted, it falls under Group A.

What You Must Know About Starches (Group B)

- Eat only one starch with each meal. For example: Do not eat rice with beans. Beans do not combine with corn or wheat tortillas, French fries (potatoes) do not combine with a sandwich (wheat), yet pasta combines with bread, pizza and/or lasagna, because they are derived from the same starch – wheat.
- Starches, if not prepared with fat (butter/oil), can be combined with sweet fruits and fresh cheeses (Group C) i.e. toast with cheese and watermelon juice.
- If you want to lose weight, cut down on your starch consumption, especially refined grains.

How to Eat Sweet Fruits and Fresh Cheeses (Group C)

- All sweet fruits combine with each other and one food from Group B (Starches), if not prepared with fat, such as butter.
- Use dates, honey, and raisins as a way to satisfy your sweet tooth.
- Dried sweet fruits also combine with fresh sweet fruits, i.e. dried pears/papaya/grapes, etc.
- When mixing sweet fruits (Group C) with raw bananas (Group E) remember to not eat starches (Group B), because they don't combine with bananas.

- Have fun experimenting with various sweet fruit combinations for juice blends and smoothies.
- You can juice the fruits or eat them in their natural state. In many cases, if you extract and consume only the vitamin-rich juice you will increase the nutritional value of the meal.

How to Eat Acidic Fruits (Group D)

- Never mix one kind of acidic fruit with any another food, including other acidic fruits.
- Eat enough at one sitting to hold you over until the next meal.
- Do not eat acidic fruits that have been dried, i.e. peaches, pineapples, apricots, oranges, berries, etc., since they are often sweetened in the process. However, if they are naturally dried with no sweetener of any kind, then, they may be eaten by themselves.
- It's always better to eat acidic fruits for breakfast, since that will ensure complete digestion of your last meal.
- It's best not to eat acidic fruits more than two times a week.

Bananas for Sure! (Group E)

- Extremely nutritious, easy to find, and full of healthy benefits.
- Raw bananas combine with all sweet fruits (Group C) when fresh.
- They combine with milk, but not with cereal (Group B).
- A meal of only bananas (or any other single fruit) will help you lose weight.
- Cooked or fried bananas combine with meats and vegetables (Group A) and one starch (Group B).

Does Milk do Your Body Good? (Group F)

- Milk is beneficial only for children during their growing years.

- Once you reach adulthood, the less milk you drink, the better.

- Milk combines with bread, butter, and cheese; with cereal; or bananas.

- Don't drink milk with meats or vegetables (Group A) or with fruits (Groups C and D).

The Gracie Diet 14-Day Meal Plan

I realize that most of these meals will be completely new to you and may seem unfamiliar, unappetizing, or even intimidating. I urge you to try each of them before you pass judgment on the Diet. View the experience as a visit to a new place or learning a new language. Approach the Diet with curiosity and an open mind. It will take a bit of practice, but the benefits are worth it. The habit of eating with a wholesome purpose will put you, your children, and your loved ones on a new path toward health and happiness.

The following 14-day plan is a good place to start. It contains recipes that the Gracie family has used for many years. They're delicious and easy to prepare. I have prepared all of them by myself many times. If I can do it, so can you! At our house we usually eat at least one sweet meal (Group C), often two, each day. We've arranged our lives so that we eat our primary cooked meal (Group A) for lunch. Since the body's metabolism is more active during the day, this makes the cooked meal easier to digest. I realize that for many families having the primary cooked meal during the day is unfeasible due to school, work and other scheduling conflicts, so they have their main Group A meal at night instead.

That is not a problem.

Following are samples of meals that adhere to the Gracie Diet combination guidelines. As you experiment with these meals, you can substitute one food for another of the same group, or you can add another food to the meal so long as it doesn't violate a combination principle for that particular group. Some meals will be familiar to you and some will be completely new. Although eating a variety of foods is best, if you find a set of breakfasts, lunches, and dinners that you take a particular liking to, you can repeat them as often as you'd like. Just don't eat the same food within 24 hours.

Experiment with these meals, develop new tastes, appreciate the variety and flexibility, but most of all understand that they will improve your health. Imagine that you are a VIP guest on some exotic island for a two-week vacation and this is what your hosts served you each day. Rejoice!

	BREAKFAST	LUNCH
MON	Oatmeal (**B**) and raisins, dates or honey (**C**) and apple juice (**C**).	**Salad:** Lettuce, broccoli, avocado, radish, onions, beats, cucumber, celery, bell peppers, hearts of palm, sprout, arugula, etc.(**A**). Olive oil and salt only. Add cashews, walnut, Brazil nuts, macadamia, etc.(**A**).
TUE	Bananas (**E**) blended with can-taloupe juice (**C**); a teaspoon of cream cheese (**C**) is optional.	**Salad:** Same as above
WED	Eggs (**A**), whole grain toast (**B**), and butter (**A**) with coffee/tea (neutral); no sugar or lemon, artificial sweetener OK.	**Salad:** Same as above
THUR	Mangos (**D**); peel, suck the juice, and spit out the pulp.	**Salad:** Same as above
FRI	Bananas (**E**) blended with watermelon juice (**C**).	**Salad:** Same as above
SAT	Vegetable Juice (see page 123) with avocado (**A**) on toasted sourdough/whole grain bread (**B**).	**Salad:** Same as above
SUN	Oranges (**D**) juiced; or peel them, suck the juice, and spit out the pulp.	**Salad:** Same as above

14-DAY MEAL PLAN

LUNCH	DINNER
Entrée: Baked salmon with rosemary (**A**), quinoa (**B**), and cream of spinach - use quinoa flour (**A-B**). **Drink:** Regular or sparkling water (no lemon), coconut water (neutral), or carrot juice (**A**); adding some of the salad ingredients (**A**) to the juice is optional.	Watermelon juice (**C**), cottage cheese (**C**), rye bread (**B**); raisins, dates, or honey (**C**) are optional.
Entrée: Chicken stroganoff (**A**), brown rice (**B**), and onion quiche - use rice flour (**A-B**). **Drink:** Same as above	Vegetable Juice (see page 123) with avocado (**A**) on toasted sourdough/whole grain bread (**B**).
Entrée: Fish soufflé (**A**), whole wheat pasta (**B**), and steamed/cooked vegetables (**A**). **Drink:** Same as above	Apple juice (**C**), cottage cheese (**C**), and rye crackers (**B**); raisins, dates or honey (**C**) are optional.
Entrée: Corn soup (**A**) and grilled Monterey Jack cheese (**A**) on sourdough/whole grain bread (**B**). **Drink:** Same as above	Honeydew melon juice (**C**), cream cheese (**C**), and whole grain crackers (**B**).
Entrée: Baked fish a la coconut (**A**), brown rice (**B**), and eggplant quiche - use rice flour (**A-B**). **Drink:** Same as above	Sweet pears (**C**); raisins, dates, or honey (**C**) are optional.
Entrée: Round roast (**A**), whole wheat pasta (**B**), and cream of corn - use wheat flour (**A-B**). **Drink:** Same as above	Cantaloupe pieces (**C**), sweet grapes (**C**), cottage cheese (**C**), and bananas (**E**).
Entrée: Shrimp (**A**) and potato (**B**) combo, potato chips/ French fries (**B**), and steamed/sautéed vegetables (**A**). **Drink:** Same as above	Fresh figs (**C**), cottage cheese (**C**), and honey (**C**).

WEEK 1

GRACIE DIET

	BREAKFAST	LUNCH
MON	Milk (**F**) and grilled Monterey Jack cheese (**A**) on sourdough/whole grain bread (**B**).	**Salad:** Lettuce, broccoli, avocado, radish, onions, beats, cucumber, celery, bell peppers, hearts of palm, sprout, arugula, etc.(**A**). Olive oil and salt only. Add cashews, walnut, Brazil nuts, macadamia, etc.(**A**).
TUE	Bananas (**E**) blended with honeydew melon juice (**C**).	**Salad:** Same as above
WED	Papaya (**C**), cream cheese (**C**); raisins, dates, or honey (**C**) are optional.	**Salad:** Same as above
THUR	Sweet pears (**C**), cottage cheese (**C**); raisins, dates, or honey (**C**) are optional.	**Salad:** Same as above
FRI	Bananas (**E**) blended with apple juice (**C**).	**Salad:** Same as above
SAT	Tangerines (**D**); peel them, suck the juice, and spit out the pulp.	**Salad:** Same as above
SUN	Milk (**F**) blended with bananas (**E**).	**Salad:** Same as above

14-DAY MEAL PLAN

LUNCH	DINNER
Entrée: Grilled chicken (**A**), quinoa (**B**), and zucchini quiche - use quinoa flour (**A-B**). **Drink:** Regular or sparkling water (no lemon), coconut water (neutral), or carrot juice (**A**); adding some of the salad ingredients (**A**) to the juice is optional.	Red apples (**C**), papaya (**C**), cottage cheese (**C**), and bananas (**E**).
Entrée: Grilled halibut (**A**), baked potatoes (**B**), and steamed/sautéed vegetables (**A**). **Drink:** Same as above	Persimmons (**C**) and cottage cheese (**C**); rye crackers (**B**) are optional.
Entrée: Squash soup (**A**) and grilled Monterey Jack cheese (**A**) sandwich on sourdough/whole grain bread (**B**). **Drink:** Same as above	Sweet grape juice (**C**), cream cheese (**C**), and whole grain toast (**B**).
Entrée: Fish soufflé (**A**), brown rice (**B**), and sautéed green beans (**A**). **Drink:** Same as above	Vegetable Juice (see page 123) with avocado (**A**) on toasted sourdough/whole grain bread (**B**).
Entrée: Onion quiche - use wheat flour (**A-B**), whole wheat pasta (**B**), and cream of spinach - use wheat flour (**A-B**). **Drink:** Same as above	Watermelon juice (**C**), Monterey Jack cheese – not melted (**C**), and whole grain crackers (**B**).
Entrée: Baked fish a la coconut (**A**), brown rice (**B**), and steamed/sautéed vegetables (**A**). **Drink:** Same as above	Cantaloupe juice (**C**), blended with pure açaí (**C**), and honey or dates (**C**).
Entrée: Steak (**A**), mashed potatoes (**B**), and corn on the cob (**A**). **Drink:** Same as above	Honeydew melon juice (**C**), cream cheese (**C**), and whole grain crackers (**B**).

WEEK 2

Parting Comment

Efficiency in combat is what has put my family on the map, efficiency in health and nutrition is what made it possible. The healthy lifestyle taught to me by my uncle and father is the greatest gift I ever received, and it is, without a doubt, the greatest gift I have ever given my children. I am happy to finally share with you the only self-defense system greater than Gracie Jiu-Jitsu, the Gracie Diet. Like any street fight, the fight for optimum health will not be an easy one. Things will not always go according to plan, and undoubtedly, you will get hit. As long as you can remain focused, stay strong, and stick to the plan, victory is yours!

Points to Remember:

- *As you start the Gracie Diet, know that it has worked for thousands of people and will work for you.*

- *If you follow the Diet 100% for two weeks, your body will be so fine-tuned that you will notice when a violation occurs.*

- *Even if you decide not to stick with it, give it a try. "The worst kind of blind individual is the one who chooses not to see." (Brazilian proverb)*

 THE GRACIE DIET IN A NUTSHELL

- *Walk or have some physical activity regularly.*
- *Sun bathe at a healthy time, and wear sunscreen.*
- *Drink a glass of water every day as soon as you wake up.*
- *Flexibility will keep you young. Stretch every day.*

ENTRÉES MENU INDEX

ONION QUICHE

Ingredients:

5 large onions sliced thin
1 tablespoon of butter
½ teaspoon of oregano
½ cup of water (4 oz)
1 package of cream cheese (8 oz)
2 teaspoons of minced parsley
2 tablespoons of chopped black olives
3 tablespoons of grated Parmesan cheese
3 egg whites (whipped to stiff peak or "snow")
240 grams (8 oz) of wheat flour*
200 grams (7 oz) of margarine or butter
Salt to taste

Servings: 4-6 people.

Making the filling:

a) In a pan, mix the butter, onions, oregano, and salt. Cook it for
   5 minutes and let it cool down.
b) In a blender mix the cream cheese and the water. In a glass
   bowl pour the mixture of water and cream cheese, and add the
   parsley, olives, and Parmesan cheese.

Making the dough:
In a medium-size baking dish, place the wheat flour* and the butter. Mix everything until the dough is smooth and even (the dough should have the consistency of damp beach sand).

Preparation:
Cover the baking dish with the dough spreading it evenly on the bottom and sides. Then add the onions (a), spreading it on top of the dough (make sure the onion filling is cold or it will dissolve the dough). Add the whipped egg whites to the cream cheese mixture (b), mixing it gently and pour everything on top of the onions. Cook in oven preheated at 350° for approximately 40 minutes. When it is golden brown, it's ready.

*This pie can also be made with rice or quinoa flour, in which case, for the same amount of flour 2 cups (16 oz /240 grams) you use less margarine or butter (5 oz /150 grams).

*Remember to use only one kind of flour/starch per meal.

ZUCCHINI QUICHE

Ingredients:
7 small zucchinis cut in thin and wide slices
½ cup of minced black olives (4 oz)
1 cube of vegetable broth
½ onion minced
3 cloves of garlic minced
1 tablespoon of olive oil
240 grams (8 oz) of wheat flour*
200 grams (7 oz) of margarine or butter

Servings: 4-6 people.

Making the filling:
Sauté the garlic and onion in the olive oil, add the vegetable broth, the zucchinis, and the olives. Let it cook for 10 minutes. Remove from stove and let it cool.

Making the dough:
Combine wheat flour and butter. Mix it until the dough is smooth and even (the dough should have the consistency of damp beach sand), then spread it in a medium baking pan and let it bake in a preheated oven at 350° for approximately 30 minutes.

Preparation:

When the dough is baked, pour the filling into it. Sprinkle a bit of grated Parmesan cheese on top and place the dish back in the oven for 5 minutes. It's done.

*This pie can also be made with rice or quinoa flour, in which case, for the same amount of flour (2 cups or 240 grams) you use less margarine or butter (5 oz or 150 grams).

*Remember to use only one kind of flour/starch per meal.

EGGPLANT QUICHE

Ingredients:
2 eggplants chopped
½ green bell pepper minced
½ red bell pepper minced
½ onion minced
3 cloves of garlic minced
2 tablespoons of minced chives
3 tablespoons of olive oil
2 tablespoons of Parmesan cheese
2 egg whites (whipped to stiff peak or "snow")
240 grams (8 oz) of wheat flour*
200 grams (7 oz) of butter

Servings: 4-6 people.

Making the filling:
Sauté the onion and the garlic in olive oil in a saucepan. When done, add the bell peppers, the eggplants, and salt. After it is cooked, add the chives. Turn the heat off, and let it cool down.

Making the dough:
Combine wheat flour and butter. Mix until the dough is smooth and even (the dough should have the consistency of damp beach sand). Then, spread it on the baking dish and bake it in a preheated oven at 350° for approximately 30 minutes.

Preparation:
When the dough is baked, pour the filling, cover it with the whipped egg whites and sprinkle the Parmesan cheese on top. Bring it back to the oven for 10 more minutes and it is ready!

*This pie can also be made with rice or quinoa flour, in which case, for the same amount of flour (2 cups or 240 grams) you use less margarine or butter (5 oz or 150 grams).

* *Remember to use only one kind of flour/starch per meal.*

CREAM OF SPINACH

ENTRÉES MENU INDEX

Ingredients:
1 bunch of spinach
½ onion minced
3 cloves of garlic minced
1 glass of water (8 oz)
½ package of cream cheese (4 oz)
1 tablespoon of olive oil
2 tablespoons of flour* (wheat, rice, or quinoa)
Salt to taste

Servings: 2-4 people.

Preparation:
Wash the spinach well and divide it in two parts.
In the blender, mix the water, cream cheese, half of the spinach, and the flour*. Chop up the rest of the spinach very small. Sauté the garlic and onion with the olive oil and add the mixture from the blender. Keep stirring until it thickens. Add the chopped spinach and cook for a couple more minutes. Serve it hot.

Remember to use only one kind of flour/starch per meal.

CREAM OF CORN

Ingredients:
2 cans of corn (washed) or 4 ears of corn
3 cloves of garlic minced
2 tablespoons of olive oil
½ package of cream cheese (4 oz)
1 pinch of nutmeg
1 cup of water (8 oz)
2 tablespoons of flour* (wheat, rice, or quinoa)
Salt to taste

Servings: 2-4 people.

Preparation:
In the blender, mix 2 cans of corn, water, cream cheese, and flour*.
Sauté the garlic in the olive oil and add the corn blend and season
with salt and nutmeg. Keep stirring until it thickens. Serve it hot.

Remember to use only one kind of flour/starch per meal.

CHICKEN STROGANOFF

Ingredients:

2 lbs of boneless chicken breast cut in small squares
1 onion minced
4 cloves of garlic minced
1 tablespoon of olive oil
1 cube of chicken broth
½ cup of water (4 oz)
¼ teaspoon of oregano
3 bay leaves
4 tablespoons of tomato sauce
½ package of cream cheese (4 oz)
½ teaspoon of dried basil
1 cup of sliced mushrooms
Salt to taste

Servings: 2-4 people.

Preparation:

Marinate the chicken breast overnight with garlic, oregano, bay leaves, and salt, in a covered glass bowl. In a saucepan, heat up the olive oil and sauté the chicken pieces. Add the onion, the chicken broth, and basil. Let it cook. Separately, mix the water*, cream cheese, and tomato sauce. It should become like a cream. Add the mushrooms to the chicken**, and let it cook. Lastly, remove the bay leaves***, add the cream cheese mixture. Mix well. Do not let it boil. It's ready.

*Tip: Don't add too much water to the chicken so the cream
  doesn't get watered down.
**Tip: We can use the same process to make meat or shrimp
stroganoff.
***Tip: Do not use oregano on fish and always remove the bay
leaves before serving.

NOTE: *This dish combines with any starch because it does not
contain any flour.*

CHAYOTE SQUASH SOUFFLÉ

Ingredients:

3 chayote squash, peeled and sliced in thick slices

½ small onion minced

3 cloves of garlic minced

1 teaspoon of oregano

2 tablespoons of olive oil

½ package of cream cheese (4 oz)

3 tablespoons of water

3 egg yolks

3 egg whites (whipped to stiff peak or "snow")

2 tablespoons of grated Parmesan cheese

Salt to taste

Servings: 2-4 people.

Preparation:

Sauté the garlic and the onion in the olive oil; Add the chayote squash, salt, and oregano and let it cook. After it is cooked, let it cool down. Mix in the blender the cream cheese, the Parmesan cheese, the egg yolks, and 3 tablespoons of water. Mix this with the chayote squash. Pour the egg whites and mix it gently. Place it all in a Pyrex baking dish greased with butter. Place it in the oven for approximately 40 minutes until golden brown. Serve hot.

NOTE: *This dish combines with any starch because it does not contain any flour.*

BAKED FISH A LA COCONUT

Ingredients:
5 fish fillets, seasoned with salt only (any mild fillet such as orange roughy, halibut, sole, tilapia, etc.)
1 large onion cut in slices
2 tablespoons of capers
2 tablespoons of minced cilantro
2 tablespoons of olive oil
13 oz of coconut milk (400 ml)

Servings: 2-4 people.

Preparation:
In a Pyrex dish mix half of the onion, half of the capers, and half of the cilantro. Place the fish fillets in the Pyrex dish and cover the fish with the rest of the ingredients. Pour in the olive oil and the coconut milk. Allow it to bake at 350° for approximately 30 minutes or until the fish is golden brown. Serve it hot.

NOTE: This dish combines with any starch because it does not contain any flour.

BAKED SALMON
WITH ROSEMARY (OR CAPERS)

Ingredients:
1 fillet of salmon (8 oz) seasoned with salt
3 cloves of garlic minced
3 rosemary leaves (or 1 tablespoon of capers)
2 tablespoons of olive oil

Servings: 1-2 people.

Preparation:
Mix the ingredients to make a pesto-like sauce (the quantity will vary according to the size of the salmon fillet). Be generous with the garlic and the rosemary (or capers). Spread the paste over the whole fish. Wrap the fish in aluminum foil and bake for 30 minutes at 350°. Serve it hot.

NOTE: This dish combines with any starch because it does not contain any flour.

FISH SOUFFLÉ

Ingredients:
4 fish fillets (salmon, orange roughy, or tilapia)
½ of a green bell pepper minced
½ of a red bell pepper minced
1 small onion minced
3 cloves of garlic minced
2 tablespoons of olive oil
2 tablespoons of minced cilantro
1 package of cream cheese (8 oz)
3 egg yolks
3 egg whites (whipped to stiff peak or "snow")
Salt to taste

Servings: 2-4 people.

Preparation:
Cook the fish in the olive oil with garlic, onion, bell peppers, and salt. Let the fish cook in its own water; do not add water. When cooked, add the cilantro. Allow it to cook until the water dries up. Mash the fish with a fork so it will crumble. Let it cool down. Whip the cream cheese with the egg yolks and 3 tablespoons of water; add this cream to the mashed fish and mix everything. Add the whipped egg whites and mix gently. Pour everything in a Pyrex dish greased with butter and bake it in a preheated oven at 350° for approximately 40 minutes or until golden brown. It's ready to serve.

NOTE: This dish combines with any starch because it does not contain any flour.

Ingredients:
1 lb of potatoes
2 eggs
½ package of cream cheese (4 oz)
¼ cup of water (2 oz)
1 tablespoon of minced cilantro
3 tablespoons of grated Parmesan cheese
1 lb of clean shrimp
2 tablespoons of olive oil
1 onion minced
2 cloves of garlic minced
2 tomatoes peeled and minced
½ green bell pepper minced
200 ml of coconut milk (7 oz)
2 tablespoons of potato starch diluted in 200 ml of water (7 oz)
Salt to taste

Servings: 2-4 people.

Preparing the potatoes:
Cook the potatoes. When done mash the potatoes and mix in
the eggs and the cilantro. In a blender mix the water and cream
cheese. Add the cream cheese blend to the mashed potatoes and
mix well. Let it sit.

Preparing the filling:

Sauté the garlic and the onion in olive oil; add the bell pepper and the tomato and let it cook for 5 minutes. Add the shrimp seasoned with only salt. Let it cook until the shrimp turn pink-colored. Add the coconut milk and the diluted potato starch to the shrimp in the pan and stir it until it thickens.

Assembling it:

In a Pyrex dish greased with butter, spread half of the mashed potato mix evenly. Pour the shrimp and then cover it with the rest of the potato mix. Sprinkle the Parmesan cheese and bake it in a preheated oven at 350° for 30 minutes and it will be ready to serve.

NOTE: Since potato is the starch of choice for this meal, French fries or potato chips would be OK. However, no other starch such as: breads, beans, rice, corn flour, etc. (Group B).

CORN SOUP

ENTRÉES MENU INDEX

Ingredients:
1 dozen ears of sweet corn
Olive oil
Salt to taste
Observation: You'll need a juicer for this one.

Servings: 1-2 people.

Preparation:
Shuck the corn and shave the kernels into a bowl. Put the kernels through the juicer. Put the "corn juice" into a pan and cook it on a low flame stirring nonstop with a wooden spoon so the corn juice does not get stuck to the bottom of the pan. When it starts to boil, it's done. Add olive oil and salt to taste.

NOTE: *You can complete this meal with a grilled Monterey Jack cheese sandwich on sourdough or whole grain bread.*

MASHED POTATOES

Ingredients:
5 medium potatoes
1 tablespoon of butter
¼ package of cream cheese (2 oz)
¼ glass of water (2 oz)
Salt to taste

Servings: 2-4 people.

Preparation:
Peel and cook the potatoes. Blend the cream cheese and the water. After cooked, mash the potatoes well and add the butter, the blended cream cheese, and salt. It's ready. Enjoy!

NOTE: *You may eat mashed potatoes (Group B) with meat, poultry, or fish, and/or vegetables (Group A).*

ENTRÉES MENU INDEX

ROUND ROAST

Ingredients:
1 (4 ½ pound) round roast
1 onion chopped
3 garlic cloves minced
1 medium carrot
½ teaspoon of oregano
3 bay leaves
4 tablespoons of olive oil
2 glasses of water (8 oz each)
Salt to taste

Servings: 4-6 people.

Preparation:
Wash the meat and place it in a glass bowl with onions, garlic, oregano, bay leaves, and salt. Poke a hole through the meat with a knife and stick the carrot in it. Cover the bowl and let it marinate for at least 8 hours in the refrigerator.

Heat up the olive oil in a pan and place the meat in it. (Wipe off the ingredients with your hand before placing the meat in the hot oil; the carrot stays in.) Move the roast around the pan until it acquires an even color all over it. Then, place the ingredients back into the pan with the meat (except for the bay leaves) and let them cook a little to a brown color; it will add flavor. Then add the water and let it cook for about 45 minutes, turning the roast once in a while. Make sure the water does not dry out completely. If you need to add a bit more, it's OK. By scraping the bottom of the pan once in a while with a wooden spoon, you will end up with the cooked ingredients and the meat juice as a flavorful sauce for the roast.

NOTE: *This dish would combine with any one starch: rice, pasta, potato, etc., (Group B) and any vegetable (Group A).*

THE RENERGY SANDWICH

*Many people wonder where my son, Rener, gets his energy from…
here is the answer.*

Ingredients:
½ ripe avocado
2 slices of whole grain wheat bread
1 scoop of almond butter
1 tablespoon of olive oil
½ bunch of spinach
Salt to taste

Servings: 1 person.

Preparation:
Wash the spinach well, and then sauté it in the olive oil. Toast
the bread, and then spread the almond butter on one piece.
Peel the avocado and spread it on top of the almond butter.
Finally, place the sautéed spinach on top of the avocado and
cap the sandwich with the other slice of toast. Try it with all the
ingredients, and then adapt it to your own preferences. If one isn't
enough, make two.

RYRON'S VEGETABLE JUICE

When my oldest son, Ryron, became a vegetarian, he fell in love with this juice.

Ingredients:
1 oz. of ginger
1 bunch of Kale
5 radishes
3 sticks of celery
1 bunch broccoli
1 bell pepper
1 cucumber
5 carrots

Servings: 1-2 people.

Preparation:
Wash all vegetables thoroughly, using any of the vegetable wash products readily available. Peel the cucumber, the ginger, and the carrots, and then pass all the vegetables through a juicer. Feel free to add additional vegetables to the mix or modify the proportions to your liking.

Also from the Gracie Family:

Gracie Jiu-Jitsu - The Master Text
Written by Grand Master Helio Gracie, this 8.5 x 11 inch, 275-page, hardbound, full-color masterpiece covers the legacy and the techniques of the Gracie Family more comprehensively than any other publication. Packed with over 1,200 detailed instructional photos, this book guides you step-by-step through the most important standing and ground techniques of Gracie Jiu-Jitsu, presented by the man who created them. For more information on the family, visit *www.GracieAcademy.com*.

Gracie Combatives®
Originally developed for the U.S. Army, Gracie Combatives is a self-defense program designed to take any person - regardless of age, gender, or athletic ability - from no knowledge to "street ready" in the the least amount of time possible. Based on the 36 most effective techniques of Gracie Jiu-Jitsu, this program can be learned from home via DVD or online streaming videos. To get started with the first three lessons for free, log on to *www.GracieUniversity.com*.

Gracie Bullyproof ®
Gracie Bullyproof is the at-home empowerment program that teaches parents how to empower their children with the verbal strategies to stand up to bullies with unshakable confidence and a series of non-violent self-defense techniques to keep them safe if they are physically attacked. The program has been featured on CNN, NBC, and Oprah.com as an effective counter-measure to bullying. Gracie Bullyproof is accessible on DVD and in online streaming video format. To watch the Parent Preparation Course for free, log on to *www.GracieKids.com*.

Women Empowered®
This comprehensive 15-lesson self-defense program for women is based on the proven verbal, physical, and psychological defense strategies taught at the Gracie Jiu-Jitsu Academy for nearly two decades. The program is available on DVD, via online streaming video, or at Gracie Certified Training Centers around the world. To watch the Women Empowered introduction for free, log on to *www.GracieUniversity.com*.

If you have any questions that are not covered in this book, or you'd like to see video tutorials on several Gracie meals and recipes, please visit:
www.GracieDiet.com